SOAP MAKING
FOR BEGINNERS

Make Natural, Fantastic Smelling Soaps Right in
Your Own Kitchen!

(Hot Process Soaps, Liquid and Melt & pour
Techniques)

Elizabeth Nol

Published by Oliver Leish

Elizabeth Nolan

All Rights Reserved

Soap Making for Beginners: Make Natural, Fantastic Smelling Soaps Right in Your Own Kitchen! (Hot Process Soaps, Liquid and Melt & pour Techniques)

ISBN 978-1-77485-081-7

Legal & Disclaimer

The information contained in this book is not designed to replace or take the place of any form of medicine or professional medical advice. The information in this book has been provided for educational and entertainment purposes only.

The information contained in this book has been compiled from sources deemed reliable, and it is accurate to the best of the Author's knowledge; however, the Author cannot guarantee its accuracy and validity and cannot be held liable for any errors or omissions. Changes are periodically made to this book. You must consult your doctor or get professional medical advice before using any of the suggested remedies, techniques, or information in this book.

Upon using the information contained in this book, you agree to hold harmless the Author from and against any damages, costs, and expenses, including any legal fees potentially resulting from the application of any of the information provided by this guide. This disclaimer applies to any damages or injury caused by the use and application, whether directly or indirectly, of any advice or information presented, whether for breach of contract, tort, negligence, personal injury, criminal intent, or under any other cause of action.

You agree to accept all risks of using the information presented inside this book. You need to consult a professional medical practitioner in order to ensure you are both able and healthy enough to participate in this program.

Table of Contents

Introduction

Many of us have often dreamed about making our own soap either because we have a specific scent in our heads that we'd like to clean our bodies with, or because buying good soap is so expensive when you can make entire batches of it at home fairly inexpensively. Perhaps it's just the satisfaction of making your own soap that appeals to you.

However, despite the fact that people have made their own soap since the beginning of recorded human history many of us also have it in our heads that making soap is difficult or even dangerous.

The truth is that making soap is as difficult and dangerous as you choose to make it. Some cold methods for making soap are as trying as making a cake and with some gloves and a pair of goggles you'll be perfectly safe to make large batches of good quality soap.

Other methods are more involved and require treating soap ingredients at high temperature and involve more risk. Some variations of these methods might not even be suitable for home use, but even here it's usually not too difficult to make the soap safely at home.

Chapter 1: One Step At A Time – Perfect Soap Making

MELT AND POUR PROCESS

If you are a newbie or just don't want to put too much effort in soap making, then I suggest you go with the "melt and pour process". This one requires a premade soap base and essential oils, herbs or colorants, depending on what you want.

Tools and ingredients you need:

A bowl that can be put in the microwave

Plastic wrap

Spoon or rubber spatula

Premade soap base (you can get it at the craft store – goat's milk, glycerin or shea butter)

Molds (go with the silicone molds)

Herbs, essential oils, colors, or/and fragrance

First, you need to put a premade soap base in a heat resistant bowl and cover a bowl with plastic wrap. This will prevent the soap from drying out in the microwave. Then, place the bowl in the microwave and melt the soap for about 30-second intervals. You can stir often in order to speed up the process.

When the soap is melted completely, you need to add ingredients of your choice (whether it is essential oils, herbs, perfume or color). After that, stir the mixture until it is well combined. Note that if you use herbs, they will come out to the surface of the mixture. Also, keep in mind that you should not stir too hard otherwise there will be bubbles.

The last step is to slowly pour the mixture into molds and let the soap cool for a few hours.

When the soap is hardened, you can remove it from the molds and it is ready for use. This process is useful when you want to make soap bars quickly. Or, if you want to surprise your friends and family with lovely and unique homemade soap gifts.

COLD PROCESS

This process is for those of you who already know how to make soaps because it involves the usage of lye, which is caustic so you have to be careful with it. This process is the act of combining fixed oils (Olive, Coconut, or Palm) and an alkali (Lye or Sodium Hydroxide). It is ideal if you want to have complete control over what your soap is made from since you get to choose all of the ingredients. But, this process requires you to be patient and cautious. When the soap is made, it should be left for 4-6 weeks to fully cure.

When working with the lye, you have to follow safety measures, so it would be a good idea to watch some YouTube videos or read a couple of articles to steer you in the right direction. In addition, always use silicone, glass or stainless steel equipment when working with lye.

But, here are some general rules to follow.

First, you have to work in a well-ventilated room, since the lye solution omits fumes. In addition to that, make sure to keep the solution on safe, far away from kids and pets, because it is dangerous. You have to wear latex or rubber gloves, goggles, pants, long sleeves and closed-toe shoes. This is because the solution can cause burns and irritations.

Here we have a Basic "cold process" recipe, but the variations are numerous, depending on what one needs and wants.

Ingredients:

30% Coconut oil

30% Palm Oil

30% Olive oil

10% Sweet Almond Oil

Lye

Additives (herbs, essential oils, colorants...)

Water

Tools:

Silicone, wood or plastic molds

Rubber spatula

Stick blender

Heat-resistant container (aluminum containers cannot be used because aluminum will react with lye)

Thermometer

1. First, you need to weigh the lye and water in order to get the perfect amount. Then carefully and slowly add lye to the water (never try to do the other way around because that will probably kill you). You have to stir until the water is clear again. Keep in mind that you mustn't breathe the lye fumes and that the lye solution will heat up. Use another bowl for mixing oils (don't add essential oils in this part) and warm them in a pot or a slow cooker.

2. After both mixtures have cooled down to 120 degrees, slowly add the lye solution into the oils mixture.

3.Use a stick blender for blending the mixture. The blender must work continuously in order for the mixture to reach the perfect density.

4.When the soap mixture has finally reached the consistency and looks like pudding, it is time to pour it into the molds. Just to mention, in case you want to add perfume, essential oils and colorants, this is the ideal time for that, before pouring it into the molds. The colorant always goes first, and then you can add oils.

5.After you poured the mixture in the molds, leave it for two days. Then, remove the soap bars from the molds, cut, and let them cure for about 4-6 weeks.

HOT PROCESS

This process is for advanced soap makers who know what they're doing. It is similar to the cold process; the only difference is, well, it involves more cooking. Also, the soap can be used as soon as it cools down. But, you can leave for a week or two to harden.

Moreover, this process means that you will cook the soap mixture in a slow cooker or in a pot on the lowest heat so as to accelerate the saponification. After that, you can add additives.

Follow the rules for the cold process because you will also be working with lye.

What you need:

Lye

Well-ventilated room

Rubber gloves, goggles, mask, long sleeves, pants

Slow cooker (or a saucepan)

Water (distilled or tap)

Stainless steel measuring spoons

Heat-resistant glass containers

Digital Scale

Thermometer

Stick blender

Silicone spatulas

Soap molds

Litmus paper

Rubbing alcohol

1. Weigh all the ingredients. Then add oils into your slow cooker and melt them completely, but don't overheat them.

2. In a heat-resistant container add distilled water. After that, slowly add/sprinkle the lye into the water (NEVER EVER add the water into the lye). It won't take too long before the lye solution heats up, so keep eyes on it. When the lye is well combined with the water, set the mixture aside to cool. Use thermometers to check the temperatures. When the temperatures are 110 degrees F, slowly add the lye solution into your slow cooker, and stir for 15 minutes, or when the mixture starts getting consistency.

3. Cook the mixture for 3 hours at the low temperature and check it every half an hour. Also, use the pH paper in order to check the neutrality of the mixture.

4. If you want to add essential oils, perfumes, glitters or colorants, you should do that when the mixture starts to cool down.

5. Pour the solution into the molds and let it cool. Remove the soap from molds and use a knife to get nicely shaped bars. Leave the soap for a couple of days to harden.

Chapter 2: Safety First

Working With Hot Oil and Lye

When it comes to soap crafting, you do need to exercise some care. Whilst the process is fairly safe as long as you are careful, it does involve working with hot oils and lye, both of which can cause nasty accidents if you are not careful.

When soap crafting, it is better to wear clothes made of natural fibers and not to wear any jewelry.

Working with Lye

Any container that has had lye in it is not suitable to use for anything else. Be sure to mark any such containers clearly and keep them away from your normal kitchen crockery and cutlery.

You should never allow your skin to touch raw lye, lye water or soap that has just been made. Lye will react with the moisture in the skin to cause painful burns and so rubber gloves are an essential safety tool to use.

To activate the lye, you will need to dissolve it in water. It is important that you measure out the lye in a container that is only used for that purpose. It is best to use a container that you can close should you need to leave the room.

In a separate, heat-proof, preferably glass container, measure out the water required to make your lye solution and add the lye to the water.

You must always as the lye to the water and not the other way around or your mixture might explode. When making your lye solution, always measure out the water first and add the lye to that, rather than the other way round or you could risk the whole mixture exploding.

It does not stop there though, once the lye has been added to the water, the fumes produced can be toxic. You should always work in a well-ventilated room when working with lye and protect your eyes with safety goggles – should the mixture splash into your eyes it can cause permanent loss of sight.

Lye and aluminum should never come into contact with one another as the form hydrogen gas. Hydrogen gas is highly combustible. (Remember the Hindenburg?)

Use heat-safe containers. Glass is your best option but you can use plastic as long as it is a strong plastic that resists corrosion.

You will always add you lye water to your fat mixture and, when doing so, pour slowly and over the back of a spoon to prevent any of the mixture splashing out.

Working with Hot Fats

As the fats heat up and melt, they do become more dangerous to work with. Be sure to use rubber gloves to protect your hands and pot holders to hold hot handles.

Pour slowly where applicable to avoid splashes of hot fat on the skin.

General Safety Tips

Read your recipe twice before attempting it and ensure that you have all the ingredients and also that you know the order things must take and techniques involved.

It is better to have an organized workspace – measure out what you need beforehand so that you can simply reach for what you need, when you need it.

If you have small kids or pets, it is better to keep them out of your work area while making soap – accidents can happen so quickly if you turn your back.

When decanting the soap into your molds you need to take care for two reasons – first of all the lye content in the soap itself can still burn the skin and, second of all, the mixture will still be warm enough to burn the skin.

If you are using any metal molds, make sure to line them with plastic wrap.

Always carry ingredients carefully, using two hands as necessary.

It is best to cover your work surface with an old towel, reserved for the purpose.

Always keep paper towels on hand to mop up any messes.

Never guess when it comes to your measurements and be sure to use accurate measuring cups, jugs, scales, etc.

If there any fat fires in the kitchen, cover with a dishtowel so that the oxygen supply is cut off. Throwing water on them will only spread the fire faster.

The soap should be kept out of the reach of children and animals while it is still curing.

If any lye is ingested, get to the nearest emergency room as fast as possible.

The fats and lye must be at the same temperature before being combined – use two thermometers to be absolutely sure.

If you want to, you can buy pH testing strips at the drugstore to ensure that your soaps are safe to use.

Ash on the outside of the soap after curing is normal but ash in the body of the soap is not. It would be better to throw away soaps that have layers of ash in the body of the soap - it means that there was too much lye used and you will not be able to do anything to rectify this.

Never use the soaps before they have properly cured. You can be seriously burned by the lye until it is completely deactivated by the curing process.

Chapter 3: Simple Recipes To Do At Home

As you will have understood, the hydro alcoholic gel is a must, which we should all have on hand at all times of the day. However, it is very popular, especially in times of epidemics, and is sometimes difficult to obtain.

The solution? Make your own hand sanitizer!

We will show you a quick and simple recipe to make your own hand sanitizer at home.

2.1 First Recipe

We will show you a recipe, nothing could be easier. Pour all ingredients into a bowl, after mix them up. Take the following elements: rubbing alcohol, optional essential oils ready and measured out, and also aloe vera. If you don't use enough aloe gel, it will dry out the skin on your hands. This act can cause a crack or bleed.

Using a funnel, you put your hand sanitizer into the bottle of your choice, remember to label it with the words "hand sanitizer", screw the top of your bottle on tight, and use.

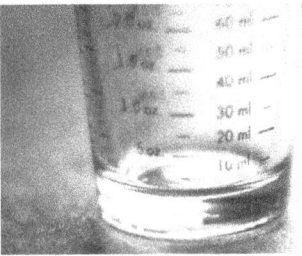

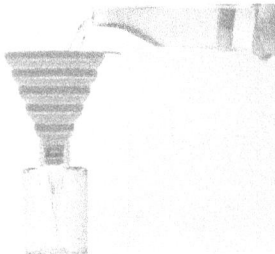

There are some tips to use hand sanitizer effectively: apply on the palm, rub your hands together and continue rubbing for 30-50 seconds. The hands will dry in 60 seconds; in this time the hand sanitizer will kill most germs.

2.2 Second recipe

Get the necessary ingredients. Some people prefer not to use alcohol in their hand sanitizers, as it has an intense smell and can have significant dehydrating effects on the skin. A witch hazel gel is a great alternative. Tea tree oil provides additional antiseptic benefits. Here there is what you will need:

-240 ml of pure aloe vera gel (preferably without additives)

-1 teaspoon and a half of witch hazel

-30 drops of tea tree oil

-5 drops of essential oil, for example lavender or mint

-Soup bowl

-Spoon

-Funnel

-Plastic container

Mix the aloe vera gel, tea tree oil and witch hazel. If the mixture seems too liquid, incorporate an additional spoonful of aloe vera to thicken it. If it is too thick, add another spoonful of witch hazel.

Incorporate the essential oil, Since the smell of tea tree oil is already quite intense in itself, do not overdo it with the added essential oils. About five drops should be enough, but if you want to increase the doses, add one drop at a time.

Pour the mixture into the container through the funnel. Place the funnel in the container and pour the hand product into it. Once filled, close it with the cap until ready to use.

If you want to take it with you during the day, opt for a small plastic squeeze bottle.

Store any leftover gel in an airtight jar.

2.3 Third recipe

We will show you an other recipe how to make the disinfectant with the WHO (World Health Organization)recipe. You need a graduated glass and scrupulously stick to the list of ingredients, without changing anything. With the doses that I will indicate you will get half a liter of disinfectant, but those who prefer can double or triple them to get more.

416 ml Ethyl alcohol

21 ml Hydrogen peroxide 3%

7 ml Vegetable Glycerin / Glycerol

55 ml Distilled water

Ethyl alcohol can be found at the supermarket in the liquor department and is colorless. I want to clarify that it is not possible to use the classic pink alcohol for this recipe. Hydrogen peroxide is easily found in any supermarket or pharmacy. You can find glycerin in the pharmacy, just ask for it at the counter! Distilled water can be bought easily from the supermarket, but if desired it can be replaced with water brought to a boil and left to cool. The procedure for making the disinfectant is very simple, just mix all the ingredients without a precise order. Transfer the liquid obtained in a well disinfected container with lid; being an alcohol-based solution this disinfectant tends to evaporate, so it is important to close it properly. Ready the disinfectant let it rest for 72 hours so it can be used! Like any disinfectant, this too must be stored in suitable containers, with a label that specifies the content and kept away from the reach of children and pets

2.4 How do you use your antibacterial solution?

There are some tips to use hand sanitizer effectively:

The first of these is not to use it on wet hands. The hydro alcoholic solution should only be used on dry hands for optimal use.

The application of the hand sanitizer must then be carried out meticulously with careful friction of at least 30 seconds:

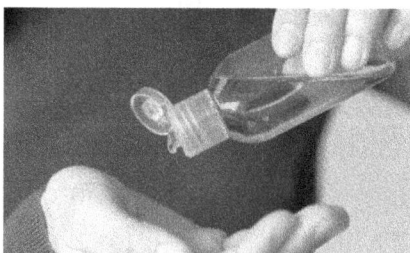

First, take a small amount of your antibacterial gel and apply it to the palm of your hand.

Then rub your hands together. At this stage, no part should be left out. Make sure to rub the back of each hand, palms, thumbs, fingertips and nails, spaces, the backs of the fingers, not forgetting the wrists.

Continue rubbing for 30 to 50 seconds. It is important to maintain a friction time with the product of at least 30 seconds until your hands are dry. If the product does not dry sufficiently, the effectiveness of the product will be reduced.

Hands generally dry; in 60 seconds during this time, the hand sanitizer will kill most germs. When your hands are dry, the process is complete. They are disinfected and do not need to be rinsed or wiped off.

2.5 Making hand sanitizer at home: Warnings

As easy as it is to make your own hand sanitizer, you should be aware that rubbing alcohol in high quantities can damage your skin. Make sure you stick to the 2:1 proportion to keep the alcohol content around 60%.

The rapid depletion of the flasks and, mixed to the high prices of the product has brought many people to make hand sanitizer at home. Working with inflammable substances may not always be a good option, especially if you haven't got any knowledge of chemistry.

Hands sanitizer mainly consists of alcohol, and hydrogen peroxide. The production of hand sanitizer could cause irritation to the eyes and narcotic effects like dizziness and nausea. You should wash your hands when you get off buses, and every time you touch something. The use of gloves could be an alternative to this.

It can prevent different infections. Another important thing to remember is that the use of hand sanitizer when your hands are dirty is not a good idea. Hand sanitizer is only an antiseptic, so on dirty surfaces the bacterium doesn't die. You have all the information you need to produce your own hand sanitizer, but you do so at your peril.

Chapter 4: You're Crash Course On Herbal Soaps

Stepping into the beauty section used to be an enjoyable experience; now it is just a confusing activity where you have to sort through a nauseating array of soaps with different purposes, sizes, colors, smells, styles and shapes. There are beauty bars, body bars, cellulite soaps, complexion soaps, exfoliating soaps, French milled soaps, glycerin soaps, handmade soaps, herbal Soaps: An Introduction soaps, milk soap, mud soaps, spa soaps, triple milled soaps, vegetable soaps, and many others.

In frustration, people just pick the brands they see on TV commercials. By doing so, they risk exposing their bodies to potentially harmful substances. If they are unsure and want to play it safe; they pick anything that says natural. But then again, it costs twice as much, plus it is probably not exactly natural per se.

The choices are endless, the ingredients are sketchy, and the budget has to be kept in mind. It is easy to be overwhelmed. How and when did something as rudimentary as soap become so totally complicated? And more importantly, how does one choose?

These "soaps" in supermarkets or beauty shops with unpronounceable ingredients are really detergents. True soaps, as in the simple suds-producing substance the ancient people and your grandmothers made in the olden days, are hard to find in your local grocery. Pure, unadulterated soap, when broken down to its simplest form, is made when a fat, either from animals or from plants and an alkali known as lye are mixed with water. True natural soaps are made when water forces the lye molecules to collide with fat molecules, resulting to two new molecules: glycerin and soap. Soap makes the suds and cleanses the body while glycerin keeps the skin moisturized. True natural soaps are ultra-rich, mild, and moisturizing.

Over time, herbs and other natural gifts offered by the earth were infused with the soaps. These herbs make the soaps healthier and more beneficial for the skin. Using herbal soaps is the perfect way to care for your skin. Herbal soaps do not only cleanse and moisturize; they also have different medicinal and therapeutic properties because of the herbs.

History of Herbal Soaps

According to legend, soap was first discovered in Mount Sapo, a hill in Rome used for animal sacrifices. Below the hill is the River Tiber, where people wash their clothes. When it rained, the rain water carried the clay-like animal fats and wood ash deposits from the sacrifices. The mixture will run down the slopes of the hill and into the river's water. One day, people realized that the clay mixed with water formed a foamy substance that helped make their laundry cleaner.

Soap, however, did not become a part of personal hygiene until the 2nd century when Galen of Pergamum, a famed physician also discovered the cleansing and medicinal properties of soaps. Before that, people rubbed flower petals, herbs, milk, oil, sand, and other items onto their bodies to remove grime, dirt, and dead skin. Many documents prove that during the time of Cleopatra, possibly even earlier, herbs were used as beauty aids, cosmetics, and cleansers. According to records, herbs and plant extracts were used by Egyptians for reddening their cheeks and lips, highlighting their eyes, massaging, and cleansing their bodies. Egyptian women used the powdered herbs' leaves and seeds on their faces, hair, and all over their bodies to make them appear more attractive, more beautiful, and fresher. Egyptians also consumed tonics made with herbal extracts and applied the oils from the herbs for massages and skin infections.

During the 14th century, as the Roman Empire began declining; bathing among other activities that focused on the body were regarded as evil. Personal hygiene deteriorated and soaps disappeared altogether. The lack of hygiene resulted into unsanitary living conditions all throughout Europe, diseases, and widespread death because of the plague.

Soap slowly began to make its comeback in many European nations as advancements in the soap making process were pioneered by French scientists. The promotion, production and use of soap slowly became common. In 1791, Nichols Leblanc patented the process of making alkali from salt and Louis Pasteur discovered the relationship between bacteria and disease a few years later.

Thus, it became necessary to fight bacteria through cleansing.

DIY Herbal Soaps

Later on in history, about 5000 years ago, Indian practitioners of Ayurveda have been encouraging the use of herbs for healthy skin and beauty. And although, the production of herbal soaps became prevalent during this period, they are only prepared in small amounts and typically produced at home using a variety of natural ingredients.

This practice of making herbal soaps in the kitchen still lives on today. Some people would rather make their herbal soaps at home because it does not only save money; it also ensures that the ingredients are natural, pure, safe, and suitable to your needs and preferences.

Chapter 5: Mixing Ingredients For Cold Process Soap

Now that you have all of your ingredients and supplies together you can start making your soap. The first thing you need to do is line your soap mold with the freezer paper making sure the shiny side will be facing the soap.

Place your stainless steel pot on your scale and zero the scale out, measure each of your solid oils zeroing out after adding each one. Place your pot on the stove on a low setting until everything melts together.

Carefully measure the lye in a bowl. You have to be careful not to get this anywhere in your kitchen because it is poison. This is why it is so important to keep your soap making supplies away from all of your cooking supplies.

Measure your water and poor it into a stainless steel bowl. The bowl you are using has to be heat resistant if it is not stainless steel. Put on your gloves and safety glasses then add the lye in the bowl with the water. Stir this together for two minutes until the water turns clear again. You will notice that there is a chemical reaction.

Hopefully since you are in the kitchen you will have some pot holders handy because you will need them to move the bowl containing the lye and water.

Next you are going to measure your liquid oils, in this case it will be your olive oil, make sure the solid oils have melted and the temperature has raised to 110 degrees. Remove the pot from the burner and turn the burner off.

Now you want to bring the temperature of you lye down to 110 degrees. You can do this by sitting the bowl in a sink with very cold water in it. Just make sure there is not so much water that it will reach the top of your bowl possible going over.

Add the liquid olive oil into the pot you mixed the solid oils in and once the temperature of the lye has cooled to 110 add it to the pot as well. While you are adding the lye into the pot you need to use the stick blender to mix it until it is completely smooth.

After about five minutes of mixing the soap will take on the texture of pancake mix. This is when you would add any fragrances or dyes but since this is a simple soap we are not going to go over that at this time.

You need to move quickly at this point because the soap has to be poured into the mold before it gets too thick. Use the cardboard box and cover the filled soap mold to help keep the heat in. Some people like to put a towel over the cardboard box but this is not necessary.

It should take about one hour from the start up until this point. After you have poured the soap in the mold you need to wash all of your tools in hot soapy water.

After your soap has sat for about 30 minutes you need to check on it. If the soap is too warm it will crack and you will need to press the crack back together with your fingers. This is why I said a towel is not really needed because this usually happens when someone uses a towel and too much heat is kept in the soap.

If you had to fix a crack in the soap after you are done cover the soap with the cardboard box. Leave the soap covered overnight and it will be ready to cut the next day.

You want to remove the soap from the mold and use the knife to score it where you want to cut it. Your knife should slide right through the soap with no problem. Next you want to stand the bars of soap on their ends inside the cardboard box so that they can dry.

You will need to allow the soap to age for about four weeks after you have cut it so put the box up in a safe place where it will not be bothered. After four weeks your soap will be ready to use.

It does take a long time for you to finally get to use your finished product but it is worth the wait. When you finally get to use your soap you will find that it lathers great and leaves your skin feeling silky smooth. If you added any essential oils you will also receive the benefits of them as well.

This soap is safe to use on all skin types and will not dry out your skin like most store bought soaps. It is great for kids and adults alike. It is also great to use in the winter instead of store bought soaps because it is so moisturizing to the skin.

If you want to keep this soap on hand just repeat the process regularly and you can store the soap in a shoe box or even plastic zip bags. It is a great alternative to using store bought soap and leaves your skin feeling clean with no nasty soap residue.

Chapter 6: Cold Process Soap

As stated before, most beginners to soap making start with cold process soaps. If this is the type of processing you'd like to try, read on to learn all about it!

Pros

• When you cold process your own soap, the entire soap is made from scratch, and you don't have to rely on pre-packaged "base soaps" to get started.

• In the same vein, you are able to control everything that goes into your soap from start to finish with this process. Don't want harsh chemicals? Don't add them!

• Cold process soap recipes are very easy to alter and tweak into your own creations. The possibilities are limitless when you use this method!

• Although it may seem daunting at first, this method is actually quite easy.

Cons

• You will be responsible for handling the lye used in the soap making process. Therefore, you may need to purchase extra items, such as protective eyewear or gloves, that you don't already own.

• This process does involve more equipment than some other methods of soap making. However, most of these tools and ingredients can be found in your kitchen already. There is a chance, though, that you will need to purchase something extra.

• This method takes a long time to finish curing. You will be waiting 2 to 4 weeks for your soap to be ready to use. If you don't have a lot of patience, or you need your soap sooner for an event, it may be best to try melt & pour or hot process soap making.

• It could be difficult to clean up after your cold process soap. You may want to designate the dishes you use for soap making only for soap purposes, since there is a high possibility that lye residue can remain on the surface of these dishes.

How-to

Are you ready to get started on your cold process soap? Then follow these easy instructions to create your first batch! Remember, this is a simple soap recipe, and you can always tweak it later, but it is best to start off slow. After you create your first successful batch, you can try different essential oils or colorants of your choice. Follow the directions carefully and you will be enjoying your first soap creation in no time!

What to gather:

Gloves, goggles, and other safety gear

Newspaper or tablecloth for covering counters

Plastic pitcher with lid

Digital scale

Stainless steel or plastic spoon

Glass or plastic measuring cup

Stainless steel pot for cooking on the stove

Immersion blender

Rubber spatula

Old towel

Soap mold of choice

Large-blade knife

Water

Lye

Canola oil

Coconut oil

Olive oil

Orange essential oil

Put on your safety gear.

First and foremost, put on your gloves, goggles, and old clothes or apron. Cover your countertops and other work space. You are about to start working with lye, and you don't want to run any unnecessary risks! Refer to Chapter 2 of this book for tips on what to do "Before You Get Started" if you need to refresh your memory on safely working with lye.

Weigh your water.

Place your plastic pitcher onto your digital scale. Zero out the scale, so that it is not including the weight of the pitcher with the weight of your water. Carefully measure out 8.5oz of distilled water in the pitcher.

Weigh your lye.

Place a glass or plastic container, such as a mason jar or plastic bowl, onto the digital scale. Zero out the scale again. Carefully open your lye and gently shake it into the container until you measure out 4oz. Immediately close the lid to the lye tightly and put it away in a safe place, out of reach of children and pets and in a location where it cannot spill.

Add the lye to the water.

Very slowly, add the lye to the water, a little bit at a time until it has been completely added. Never add the water to the lye! This can create a violent chemical reaction similar to combining baking soda and vinegar—and you definitely don't want a lye volcano in your kitchen!

Stir.

With a stainless steel or plastic spoon, stir the lye and water mixture gently until all of the lye dissolves. If it begins to steam or bubble, don't worry. That's normal! Make sure to rinse your spoon thoroughly after you finish this step.

Cool the lye-water.

Put the lid on your plastic pitcher and set it to the side. The mixture should be around 200 degrees Fahrenheit right now, and you want it to cool down to 100 degrees Fahrenheit. Set it in an out-of-the-way place where children, pets, and other members of your household cannot reach it. Be sure to label it so no one bothers it!

Weigh your oils.

Place a glass or plastic measuring cup on your digital scale and, once again, zero out the scale. Slowly measure out 12oz canola oil and set it aside. Repeat this process one at a time for 8oz coconut oil and 8oz olive oil. Remember that soap ingredients are measured by weight, not by volume, so your solid coconut oil and liquid olive oil will need to be the same weight, even though they won't be the same volume!

Melt the solid oils and liquid oils together.

Turn your stainless steel soap pot on medium heat on the stove, and begin to melt the solid oils. Stir gently as they melt, and keep cooking and stirring until they reach 110 degrees Fahrenheit. Then, turn off the heat and add the liquid oils. Stir these into the melted solids until everything is combined thoroughly.

Measure your additives for later.

Place a clean measuring cup on your digital scale and zero out the scale. Measure out 1.6oz of orange essential oil and set aside. This will be used later in the process, but you want to have it handy and measured out beforehand. Remember to do this with any additives you plan to use in your future recipes! For this first beginner recipe, orange oil is all you will need.

Add the lye-water to your oils.

For this step, you must be sure you will be uninterrupted from your soap making. You absolutely cannot leave the mixture unattended at this point!

Make sure your pot of oils and your pitcher of lye-water are both at 100 degrees Fahrenheit. Slowly and carefully begin to pour the lye-water into the pot of oils, stirring as you go.

Mix to trace.

After the lye-water has been completely added, grab your immersion blender and place it into the mixture. Turn it on for 5 seconds at a time to "pulse" the mixture. Repeat this pulsing until the mixture has completely come together and everything looks smooth. This means you have reached "trace."

Mix in additives.

Stop using the immersion blender and pour in the orange essential oil you measured out earlier. Stir it in carefully with a spoon. During this step, you would also add color, other oils, fragrances, flowerbuds, or any other ingredients you want to include in your soap. For this recipe, however, we are keeping it simple.

Pour into mold.

Line your soap mold with freezer paper. Carefully pour your soap mixture into your chosen soap mold, making sure to spread it as evenly as possible. Scrape the pot and smooth the mixture into the mold using a rubber spatula. Then, gently thump the mold against the countertop to break up any bubbles that may have formed inside the soap. Don't do this too hard, or you may splash yourself with caustic raw soap!

Let sit.

Cover the soap in the mold with a towel and set in a warm place away from the reach of children or pets. Label your soap so that anyone in your household will not bother it. Leave it alone for 48 hours.

Clean up.

While you are still wearing your protective gear, clean everything you have used for your soap making. It is still unsafe to touch the residue from this process, as it can burn or irritate your skin even now. After you have cleaned and dried everything, it is safe to remove your protective gear.

Slice soap and let cure.

After the soap has saponified for 48 hours, you can slice it with a large-blade knife however you prefer to cut it. Then, simply set it aside and let it cure! This process will generally take about 4 weeks, but it is a very important step. It will keep the soap from damaging your skin and allow it to moisturize completely.

And there you have it! You have just finished the cold process method of soap making! This simple soap recipe is a great place to start, but read on for even more exciting cold process recipes.

Example Recipes

The following example recipes will give you the ingredients and amounts needed, divided into easy to understand sections labeled Base Oils, Lye-Water, and Additives. Simply follow the directions outlined above, but substitute these ingredients instead, for fun new ways to make cold process soap!

Mean Green Exfoliant Soap

Base Oils:

10.8oz olive oil

9oz rice bran oil

7.2oz palm oil

7.2oz coconut oil

1.8oz illipe butter

Lye-Water:

4.8oz lye

12oz distilled water

Additives:

1/2 tsp green chromium oxide pigment powder

0.5oz lemongrass essential oil

0.5oz peppermint essential oil

1 tbsp poppy seeds

2 tsp ground pumice

1 tbsp walnut shell powder

Lavender Soap

Base Oils:

5.4oz coconut oil

9oz palm oil

9oz rice bran oil

3.6oz soybean oil

1.8oz grapeseed oil

3.6oz shea butter

3.6oz cocoa butter

Lye-Water:

12oz distilled water

4.8oz lye

Additives:

1oz lavender essential oil

.05oz tea tree oil

.05oz lavender flowers

1/2 tsp lavender ultramarine pigment powder

Banana Soap

Base Oils:

3lbs 1.5oz olive oil

3lbs 1.5oz coconut oil

6oz rice bran oil

4.5oz shea butter

Water-Lye:

36oz distilled water

15.6oz lye

Additives:

1 banana, unpeeled, turning brown

Peppermint Rosemary Soap

Base Oils:

3oz cocoa butter

7.2 oz soybean oil

10.8oz olive oil

8oz coconut oil

2oz almond oil

5.8oz rice bran oil

1.5oz beeswax

Water-Lye:

13oz distilled water

5oz lye

Additives:

0.8oz rosemary essential oil

0.3oz peppermint essential oil

Simple Goat Milk Soap

Base Oils:

20oz coconut oil

20oz olive oil

5oz rice bran oil

5oz avocado oil

4oz castor oil

5oz shea butter

5oz almond oil

9oz goat's milk

Water-Lye:

9oz lye

9.5oz water

Additives:

4tbsp oatmeal, dry

4tbsp honey

Chapter 7: Lye Solution

This is what I know and you are about to know about the mysterious lye solution, as this might be the first time you are hearing or rather reading about it.

A caustic chemical, that once in contact with your skin causes burns and if handled in the wrong manner, will cause serious injuries. Protect yourself when making soap to have fun and not have a nightmare when doing this.

When you make soap using cold process, you are required to use lye, which is also called Sodium Hydroxide. When dry it is Sodium Hydroxide, but when in liquid form that's when it is referred to as lye.

Other uses of lye include:

●In cleaners

• Manufacturing of drain openers.

Being that the powder is very corrosive when in liquid form, it is advisable to learn how to treat it carefully and take care of yourself in the process.

You can also purchase lye from your local supermarket if you do not want to go through the process of mixing the powder with water. Just make certain the solution you buy is made of water and Sodium Hydroxide only. Do not under any circumstance pick lye that is potentially a drain cleaner as the repercussions will be irreversible.

Things to be aware of when buying lye include:

Know the ratio of water to lye when you purchase lye. On the container, it should clearly show the ratio. It can be 50% water and 50% lye.

Purchase in large quantities of 25 to 50-pound bags. Use soap makers as your guide when purchasing lye in large quantities.

Add a lye calculator after selecting your lye type to help you measure the right amount of lye you will use in your recipe.

Liquid lye will require extra attention on the calculations. If you are not really good in math or just don't want to trouble yourself doing calculations, use Sodium Hydroxide instead. All you will do is add water according to the amount you have used.

Make sure when you buy lye, use a retail store that is reputable and not a hardware store. The possibility of getting pure and clean lye from a reputable retail store or supplier is greater than a hardware shop.

Spotting debris or black specks floating on your lye solution are an indication of impure lye product.

Below are some precautions you can follow to protect yourself, your pets and children from being harmed with coming in contact with lye:

If you store lye in plastic containers make sure they can hold the powder and not react. To test this can be through pouring hot boiling water into the container, if it holds, you can use it. DO NOT use plastics from dollar stores.

Inform your children of the dangers that can come from using lye. The earlier you warn them, the better and they will be aware of not disrupting you when you work.

Make sure you never, under any circumstance, leave lye unattended. When you are not using it, store it in containers and lock them up in secure locations.

If you have pets, let them loose outside while you work or keep them in crates to prevent them from running into you while you work or trip and spill lye on themselves or yourself.

Make certain that your container with lye has labels on it to avoid mixing or confusing them with other ingredients. Keep a spoon in the container and don't use for other purposes.

Store your lye in tight containers. Use stainless steel and not zinc or aluminum containers as lye will react with them.

When handling lye, make sure you are covered up and protected:

● This means use rubber gloves that come to your elbow

● Be in an area that is well-ventilated and wear a breathing mask.

● Use goggles that are fitting and secure around your eye area. If you have not been using it, be certain that one incident will make you blind.

- To prevent you clothes from staining, get a rubber apron that is about knee length. Also use a hairnet, just as a precaution.

Saponification

This is the chart in which you use to check the ratio of how much lye or Sodium Hydroxide you can have or add to fats that you are using. It was created by American soap-maker Elaine White.

The ratio with which you add caustic soda to oils is important as too much can burn your skin off and too little lye will mean that your soap will be rancid too fast because of the extra amount of fat in the soap.

There is a listing of caustic soda that is used for hard soap making and for liquid soap by using potassium hydroxide.

The charts below are a representation of the ratio of oils and lye can be used: The diagram is from

Table 4.1

Table 4.2

Table 4.3

There are columns in the chart displayed above (Table 4.3) that show "Soft/Hard", "Fluffy Lather", "Oil/Fat", "Skin care", "Stable Lather" and "SAP". Each of these segments is a soap characteristic and if the correct acid is used, it can be produced as categorized.

A description of what each segment means and their importance is as follows:

Hard/Soft segment; what specific acid will produce a bar of soap that is either soft or hard. A bar of soap dissolves quickly if it is too soft and ends up being mushy. A certain degree of hardness should be in your soap through a combination of soft oils and hard oils.

Fluffy Lather segment; a certain amount of a specific acid will result in the soap producing fluffy lather which is thick and bubbly yes will easily wash away.

Skin care segment; the benefit of the soap that you are producing and its effect on the skin. This is dependent on a number of vitamins used in the mixture and the moisturizing and mildness properties of the soap.

Cleansing segment; it tells how well your acid cleans. There are oils that are harsh and can lead to skin irritation. Combine oils that when saponified are harsh with those that when saponified are mild to create a soap that is well balanced between a conditioning and cleaning soap bar.

How the Saponification chart works:

From the charts above, I am going to give you an example of how to use the chart in calculating how much lye you require.

If you are making a batch soap with 1 pound of avocado oil, castor oil measuring 3 pounds and coconut oil at 4 pounds, you will calculate the amount of lye you will require for each oil then add them together to know in total how much lye you will use in your sample soap in order to saponify the oils and fats in it; (SAP values vary depending on which chart you are using)

•You calculate the SAP value of coconut which is 191.1/1000x4 pounds to get you 0.7644 pounds of lye that will saponify with the coconut oil. If you will use 8% lye discount, multiply your answer with 0.92 to get 0.7032 pounds. This is the amount of discounted lye that will completely saponify with your coconut oil.

•SAP for avocado oil i.e. 128.6/1000x1 to get 0.1337 pounds of lye. Now that answer with 0.92 to get 0.1230 pounds of discounted lye required to saponify with your avocado oil.

•SAP for castor oil, 128.6/1000x 3 to get 0.3858 pounds of lye that will saponify completely with the 3 pounds of castor oil. If you use discounted castor oil by 5%, take the 0.3858 x 0.95 to give you 0.3665 pounds of lye that will saponify completely with your castor oil.

●Now add 0.7032 + 0.1230 + 0.3665 pounds to get 1/1927 pounds of lye that you will use in your soap to saponify the oils in it.

Hope this helps you when making your soap.

Chapter 8: Soap Making Techniques

There are 4 common methods for making a bar of soap: cold process, hot process, melt and pour, and hand milling. The first two involve the use of lye, while the other two don't. Making liquid soap also requires lye.

Soap Making with Lye

When making soap using lye, you'll notice that all recipes instruct you to blend together the oil mixture and lye solution until they reach trace. This means that you'll have to blend until the two mixtures are completely mixed. If some oil remains separate, it will leave pockets of lye once transferred in the mold.

A mixture that's reached a light trace looks like a cake batter. A medium trace resembles pudding but can still be poured. A thick trace retains its shape and will likely need to be spooned to transfer into the mold.

Cold-Process Soap Making

Cold process is the method of making soap without applying any external heat to "cook" the soap. It's the most common technique used in making soap with lye.

Pros:

You can customize every ingredient according to your preference.

You can include fresh ingredients, such as milk and purees in the soap you're making because you have control over the saponification process.

You can manipulate the trace of soap batter and be more creative by making swirls, frosting, and other effects.

Cons:

Cold process soaps require at least 4 weeks to cure.

It has a finicky temperature requirement. You need to make sure that the temperatures of the oils and lye solution are within 10° of each other before mixing.

Some FD&C and mica colorants tend to morph due to the high pH environment.

How to Make Cold-Process Soap

Choose a recipe and assemble the required ingredients and safety gear. Prepare your mold.

Using a digital scale, weigh out the required amount of ingredients separately. Wear goggles and rubber gloves whenever you're handling lye.

In a well-ventilated area, slowly add lye to the water. Using a rubber spatula or a heavy-duty plastic spoon, stir until the lye is completely dissolved. As the lye dissolves, the mixture will get quite hot so you need to take precautions when handling it. Set the mixture aside and allow to cool to 100-120° F.

While the lye mixture is cooling, combine the oils in a stainless steel pot and warm them together until they're melted. You can also choose to melt the solids first before adding the liquid oils. Remove the oils from heat and allow to cool to 100-120° F.

To test the temperature, you can use an infrared thermometer every 5 to 10 minutes or place a candy thermometer in each container. If the lye solution is cooling faster, you can slow down the cooling process by placing the container in a warm water bath. If the oils are cooling faster, heat them up a bit.

Although mixtures are usually combined when they're between 100-120°F, you can mix them at the temperature of your choice. What's important is that the two mixtures are at 10° of each other.

Once both mixtures reach the desired temperatures, slowly add the lye solution to the oils. Using a stick blender, stir the mixture manually for about 30 seconds then turn the blender on and blend for another 30 seconds. Alternate until the desired consistency is achieved.

Make sure that the blade is completely submerged before turning the blender on or you'll splash the mixture everywhere. If you're adding extras such as essential oil and colorants, bring the mixture to a light trace. If not, bring it to a medium trace.

Add the extras and pulse the stick blender a few times to bring the batter to a medium trace.

With your rubber gloves still on, quickly transfer the batter into the mold. If needed, smooth the top with a wooden spoon or rubber spatula.

At this point, the soap is still caustic and can irritate your skin. If your skin touches the raw soap batter, rinse with cold water.

Insulate or freeze your soap for at least 24 hours. To insulate, cover the mold with a piece of cardboard and wrap it with a towel. If you don't want to insulate your soap, you can just leave it in the freezer.

If you choose to insulate, check the soap once in a while. If you see any cracks forming on top, the soap is too warm and you'll have to remove the cardboard and towel.

Remove the soap from the mold and slice it into bars using a knife or a wire soap cutter.

Put the soap bars on pieces of wax paper and leave them in a dry area for 4 to 6 weeks, turning occasionally. Keep an inch between bars to allow air to circulate.

Curing is a required step for all cold-process soaps. Without it, lye won't be fully neutralized and the soap will be too harsh to the skin.

Insulate or Freeze?

Insulating your cold process soap will keep its temperature high as it hardens in the mold. The main reason for doing this is to promote the gel phase—a stage in the saponification process where soap heats up to 180°F and looks gelatinous.

Forcing your soap into the gel phase will give it a more vibrant color and a slightly shiny appearance. It also prevents the formation of soda ash—a white, ashy film that can make soap feel crumbly. Gelled soaps are also easier to remove from the mold. If you use natural colorants, such as madder root powder and turmeric, your soap will have a dull look unless they undergo the said phase.

Gel phase isn't a requirement in cold process soap making. It's more of a personal preference, affecting only the appearance of soap and not its quality. In fact, if your recipe includes fruits, honey, milk, and alternative liquids, you should freeze your soap or leave it uncovered on the counter to harden. Forcing it to gel can cause an unpleasant smell and discoloration.

Your other option is to leave your soap at room temperature without cover. Depending on the temperature of the oil and lye when you mixed them and how warm the room is, your soap may gel or not. Sometimes it can go through a partial gel phase, making the color in the middle darker than the rest.

Working with Liquids Other Than Water

Water isn't the only liquid that you can mix with lye in cold-process soap making. Goat's milk is the most popular substitute for water because it makes the soap creamier and more moisturizing. Other alternatives are coconut milk, tea, buttermilk, and beer.

It still isn't established whether the moisturizing and healing properties of these water substitutes survive after reacting with lye. Even if they don't provide additional benefits, using them can add a personal touch to your handmade soap.

Liquids other than water react differently to lye. Usually, they produce more caustic steam, become foul-smelling, and turn brown. The bad smell won't stay in your cured soap but the reaction can be really nasty so you have to take extra precautions when working with any of them.

Place your container with the liquid in the sink before adding and mixing lye. Some liquids tend to bubble over and in case that happens, the solution won't spill onto the floor or counter.

Make sure that your work area has great ventilation. The fumes from the solution could be heavier and more foul smelling.

Always chill your liquid before adding the lye. It's also a good idea if you're working with just plain distilled water.

If you're working with milk, it should be partially frozen before adding the lye. Dissolve lye little by little, allowing the solution to cool down before adding more lye and keeping the temperature from exceeding 100°F.

If you're going to use a carbonated drink, such as beer, leave it on your counter for a few days, stirring frequently to make sure it's flat.

If you're working with a liquid that's high in sugar or contains alcohol, use it with a small batch of soap first to see how it would react with your other ingredients. It's also important to remember never to insulate this soap.

Work much slower than when you're using plain water.

Hot-Process Soap Making

This method of making soap is more like a variation of the cold process. Most of the steps are the same except for the added heat. The mixture is cooked in an oven or crockpot, speeding up the saponification process.

Pros:

You can customize every ingredient according to your preference.

Soap takes less time to harden than cold-process soap and can be used right away.

Clean-up is relatively easier.

Cons:

Because you're working with a thick soap batter, swirls and layers will be difficult to make.

The high temperature can cause the scent of some essential or fragrance oils to fade.

Adding fresh ingredients can be difficult since they tend to sear in the cooking process.

How to Make Hot-Process Soap

Choose a recipe and assemble the required ingredients and equipment. Prepare your mold.

Using a digital scale, weigh out the required amount of ingredients separately. Wear goggles and rubber gloves whenever you're handling lye.

In a well-ventilated area, slowly add lye to the water and stir until lye is completely dissolved. Set the mixture aside and allow to cool for about 20 minutes to 100-120° F.

Place the solid oils in the crockpot that's set on "low". Once melted, you can add the liquid oils.

If you'll be using the oven instead of the crockpot, you can do this with the stove.

When the oils are completely liquefied, turn the crockpot off and then slowly add the lye solution. Make sure that the oils are below 180°F when you add the lye solution to avoid any negative reaction.

Blend the mixture using a stick blender. Make sure that the blade is completely submerged before turning the blender on or you'll splash the mixture everywhere. Bring the mixture to a trace.

Set the crockpot on "low". Put the lid on to minimize the amount of water escaping from the pot. If you're using the oven, heat it to no more than 170°F. Place the soap mixture in an oven-proof container with lots of extra space and follow the same instructions.

Normally, you'll see bubbles rising from the edges. If lots of bubbles are forming, you can gently stir down the soap mixture. If not, you can just simply leave it to cook. While it's still cooking, scrape the crockpot's sides to reduce the amount of soap forming on the sides.

Depending on your recipe, the soap mixture will begin to appear like Vaseline in 30 minutes to an hour. You can check if it's done by taking a small sample and rubbing it between your fingers. The soap should feel waxy.

A more reliable way of testing for doneness is the tongue test. Touch the soap to your tongue. If there's a "zap" then your soap isn't fully cooked yet. Continue cooking until there's no more "zap".

If you'll be adding colorants, mix them with a little olive oil while the soap is cooking. Because your soap will be thick by the time it's cooked, the colorants won't mix well unless you pre-disperse them.

Once the soap is cooked, turn the heat off. Remove the crockpot sleeve from the heating pot. If you're adding any botanical extracts orbits, mix them in. Add fragrance or essential oils only when the soap's temperature is below 180°F. If fragrance is added when the temperature is still too high, the smell may not incorporate well into the soap. Add the colorants and mix.

It's important to work fast on this step as it will be a bit difficult to mix once the soap cools. It's also a good idea to heat all the additives slightly if they're cold before adding them to the soap.

For first-timers, it's best to add only one fragrance and color. If you're using several colors or want to make layers or a swirl of color, separate out some portions of soap. Add the pre-mixed colorants to the separated portions and quickly stir with a whisk.

Since the soap mixture is thick, you won't be able to pour it. Instead, scoop it into the mold quickly. Tap the mold filled with soap on the counter several times to get rid of any air pockets.

Cover the mold and set it aside. After 24 to 48 hours, you can cut the soap into bars. They can be used immediately or you can let them cure for a few weeks to allow extra water to evaporate and make the soap harder.

Liquid Soap Making

There are a few methods of making liquid soap and the most common follow the hot-process method of creating a soap paste. What differentiates liquid soap from hot- or cold-process soap is the type of lye it requires. Instead of sodium hydroxide (NaOH), liquid soap uses potassium hydroxide (KOH).

Pros:

If you plan on selling handmade soaps, liquid soap will be more profitable.

Cons:

The process is more complicated and requires a lot of patience.

How to Make Liquid Soap

Choose a recipe and prepare all the required ingredients and equipment. Because making liquid soap is more difficult, beginners may want to stick to a simple tried-and-tested recipe.

Using a digital scale, weigh out the required amount of ingredients separately. Wear goggles and rubber gloves whenever you're handling lye.

Place the oils in the crockpot set on low, melting the solids first before adding the liquids. Heat up the mixture to 150-170°F.

While the oils are in the crockpot, add lye to the water. If you notice a crackling sound, don't worry. It's normal for potassium hydroxide to react this way as it dissolves. Mix the solution completely and until it's clear.

When the oils are completely liquefied, slowly add the lye-water. There's no need to wait for the solution to cool first. With the stick blender still turned off, stir the lye solution and oils together.

Blend the mixture with the stick blender. Make sure that the blade is completely submerged before turning the blender on to keep the mixture from splashing everywhere. Bring the mixture to a medium trace with a pudding-like consistency. This could take up to 30 minutes, depending on the type of oils you're using.

Cover the pot with the lid. After 15 to 20 minutes, check to see if there are oils that separated. If there are, stir the mixture. Put the lid back. Check and stir the mixture every 30 minutes. It will take about 3 to 4 hours for the soap to cook.

In the time it takes to cook, the soap will transform and have different consistencies. After about 2 hours, it will become a solid taffy which is difficult to stir. Use a potato masher to break it up. Eventually, the mixture will start getting creamy.

Once the mixture has softened and become translucent, add an ounce of the soap paste to two ounces of boiling water. Stir and break up the soap until it's completely dissolved. If the liquid is a bit cloudy, the paste is ready. If it's cloudy or milky, the paste isn't cooked long enough.

It's also possible that you've made some errors in measurement.

Observe the test mixture as it cools. If it stays clear, you can continue. Boil the required amount of water and pour it to the soap paste. Stir it a bit with the potato masher or a spoon. Switch off the heat and put on the lid.

After about an hour, stir the soap some more. More likely, it's still gooey and chunky. Put the lid back on and leave it overnight to dissolve.

Once the paste has completely dissolved, you have to neutralize the soap before adding fragrance. A neutralizing solution is required as liquid soap uses about 10% more lye than bar soaps.

Turn the crockpot on and bring the liquid soap up to 180°F. While the soap is heating up, mix the required amount of neutralizing solution in a separate container. You can use a 33% Borax solution or 20% boric acid solution to neutralize the soap. To make the Borax solution, add 3 oz. of Borax for every 6 oz. of boiling water. To make boric acid, add 2 oz. of Borax for every 8 oz. of boiling water.

Prepare about ¾ ounces of this solution for every pound of soap (excluding the added water). Round down the amount of neutralizer as too much of it can make your soap cloudy.

Once the soap mixture is hot enough, add half of the Neutralizer. Stir well and observe. If it doesn't become cloudy, add the remaining half.

When soap is already neutralized, you can add fragrance, if desired. Because fragrance oils may react with liquid soap, it's best to test it first on a small amount of your finished soap.

Allow the liquid soap to cool before transferring it into large containers. Place them in a cool place and allow the soap to rest for about a week. During this time, cloudiness should clear up and insoluble solids should settle.

Transfer your liquid soap into their final containers carefully to avoid disturbing the settled solids.

Soap Making without Lye

Is it really possible to make soap without using lye? The answers are both yes and no.

Lye is essential in soap making—without it, there'll be no soap. But you can still make soap without lye. Hand milling and melt-and-pour methods allow you to make handmade soaps using pre-made soaps, so there'll be no need for you to worry about handling lye.

Melt-and-Pour Soap Making

This method is the easiest way of making soap. You only have to melt pre-made soap and add your desired fragrance.

Pros:

Soap doesn't require much time to make and can be used after it hardens, which usually takes only a few hours.

With parental control, even kids as young as 4 will be able to make soap through this method.

Soap doesn't have high pH so there's no need to worry about fragrance oils causing negative reactions.

You can make layered soap with clean and straight layers.

Cons:

Soap is prone to sweating (glycerin dew) due to the extra glycerin content.

You can't add fresh ingredients because they will eventually go bad.

Soap base can burn and if it does, it would be difficult to work with.

How to Make Melt-and-Pour Soap

Choose a recipe and assemble the required ingredients and equipment. Prepare your mold.

Measure out the required amount of melt-and-pour soap base and cut them into small chunks. Make sure that all the equipment you're using is clean. The soap will pick up any dirt, which will be difficult to remove. Place the soap base in a glass container.

Some soap makers cover their container with Saran Wrap to keep the soap from drying out. Most soaps turn out fine even without doing this so it's up to you if you want to be on the safe side.

Place the glass container in the microwave and heat the soap up 30 seconds at a time. Take the container out and stir the soap. Repeat this step until soap is completely melted.

While the soap is in the microwave, measure out the required fragrance. If you're making your own soap recipe, the rule of thumb is to add 0.4 ounces of fragrance or essential oil for every pound of soap. You can use less or more depending on how strong or light your fragrance oil is.

Once the soap is completely melted, remove it from the microwave and add the fragrance oil. If you choose to add some color, make sure that the dye you're using is soap-safe and skin-safe. Stir the melted soap gently to blend the color and incorporate the fragrance completely.

Avoid stirring too hard to prevent bubbles from forming. If there are bubbles, spray a little bit of rubbing alcohol to get rid of them.

Pour the soap into the prepared mold and cover it with Saran Wrap. Set it aside to cool and harden. It takes several hours for the soap to be ready at room temperature. If you place it in the fridge, (but never in the freezer) the soap will harden in about an hour.

Once the soap has completely hardened, it should be easy for you to remove the soap bars from the mold. If there are bars that won't pop out, run some hot water over the bottom of the mold. The bar should fall easily.

Trim off any imperfections using a small knife, if desired. You can use your finished soap immediately since the soap base is already cured.

Hand-Milling Soap

Also known as re-batching, hand-milling is the process of giving new life to soap. This method involves the grating and melting of soap that's already been made and adding fragrances, colors, or any additives you want.

Hand-milling is a great way to reuse bits of leftover soap. It also offers a way to fix a batch of soap if you made a mistake.

Pros:

You'll be able to use delicate ingredients that aren't compatible with the lye solution.

Curing soap takes at most 2 weeks.

Clean-up is super simple and easy.

Cons:

You can't add fresh ingredients because they will eventually go bad.

The high temperature can cause the scent of some essential or fragrance oils to fade.

Swirls and layers are difficult to make because you're working with thick soap batter.

How to Hand Mill Soap

The steps described below are for fixing mistakes, but you could easily adapt the steps for the reprocessing of leftover soap.

If the soap you're going to use has been curing for a few days, grate it using a cheese grater. If it's still too soft to grate or freshly made, you can just chop it into small pieces.

Place the grated soap in a glass oven dish or into a crockpot. Add some liquid and stir the mixture gently. You can use plain water or milk (goat's, cow's, or coconut milk) to melt the soap. Assuming that you're using a week-old soap, add about 2 ounces of liquid for every pound of grated soap. It if doesn't look wet enough, add another ounce. Fresher or softer soap will require less water while older ones will need more to melt.

You won't have to worry if you end up adding too much liquid. Your soap will only require more time to cure before it's ready to use.

If the mistake you're trying to fix is leaving out oil or not adding enough lye solution, you can add those at this time. Depending on the amount of lye solution you'll add, your soap may not need the liquid from the previous step. If it does, just add the liquid a little at a time.

Set your oven between 150°F and 170°F or your crockpot on low and put the lid on. If you're using the oven, make sure the dish is tightly covered.

After an hour, remove the lid and stir the mixture gently. It should be starting to liquefy and the edges should start to look translucent. Put the lid back on. Allow it to cook for another hour.

After another hour, stir the mixture up again and mash out any lumps. Let it cook some more until it's completely softened, translucent, and pourable.

Once the mixture has achieved the consistency required, add any additives that you want to incorporate into your soap and stir it up well. If you're hand-milling unscented soap, start with about ½ ounce of fragrance per pound of soap.

Scoop the soap into your prepared mold. Push it down with a rubber spatula or spoon and tap the mold on your counter so the soap settles into the mold. Set it aside for at least 24 hours.

Pop the soap out of the mold and allow it to harden completely. The amount of time your soap needs to cure depends on how much liquid you added.

Tweaking a Soap Recipe

As a beginner in soap making, it's best to stick with the recipe. But sometimes, you may want to change the percentage of one or more of the oils or the oil itself. These general guidelines should help if you choose to do so.

Do you want to increase the amount of lather or the size of your soap's bubbles?

Increase the percentage of oils that add to bubble lather, such as coconut oil, babassu oil, and palm kernel oil.

Decrease the amount of free oils (super fat) since too much of these reduce lather.

Use lather-increasing additives, such as sugar, sodium lactate, sodium citrate, or rosin.

Replace water with liquids that can boost lather, such as wine or beer.

Do you want to stabilize your soap's lather?

Use 5% to 10% of castor oil in your recipe.

Add or increase the percentage of oils and butters that contribute to lather, such as almond oil, lard, palm oil, sunflower oil, cocoa butter, or shea butter.

Decrease the percentage of oil that hinders or don't contribute much to lather, such as olive oil.

Do you want to increase conditioning in your soap recipe?

Substitute water with other liquids, such as milk, aloe vera juice, or yogurt.

Increase the super fat of total oils in your recipe.

Add or increase the percentage of nourishing oils, such as olive oil, sunflower oil, avocado oil, rice bran oil, or apricot kernel oil.

Use 5% to 10% of luxury oils, such as argan oil, flaxseed oil, jojoba oil, or hemp seed oil.

Do you want to increase the hardness of your soap?

Increase the percentage of hard oils or oils that are solid/semi-solid at room temperatures, such as coconut oil, babassu oil, palm oil, or lard.

Use 0.5% to 1% (based on total soap recipe) of stearic acid.

Use 1% to 5% of beeswax.

Add 0.5 oz. of sodium lactate for every pound of oil in your recipe.

If you decide to make some changes in the recipe (even minute ones) use a lye calculator to come up with the right amount of lye. Different types of oil need different amounts of lye to turn into soap. Not using the right amount of lye can make your soap either too soft or too harsh.

Using a Lye Calculator

There are several free online lye calculators you can use if you have to make some changes in the soap recipe. The most common of which is SoapCalc.

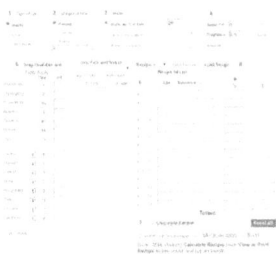

Don't be intimidated with all the empty boxes and the values that you have to enter. Using a lye calculator isn't as hard as it looks.

Select the Type of Lye that you'll be using. The default is NaOH, which as you already know is the lye for making bar soaps.

Select the unit of measure (Pounds, Ounces, or Grams) for the Weight of Oils in your recipe. Enter the total weight of oils in your recipe in the box below. Remember that this weight excludes essential oils and fragrance oils.

Water refers to the amount of water that you'll be using. The default is Water as % of oils with a value of 38. As a beginner, it's best to stick with this option since this is what's recommended for those who are just starting out. Decreasing the percentage of water in your recipe will make your soap reach trace faster.

Super Fat refers to the percentage of oils that won't be transformed into soap but will remain in the soap. The default value is 5%, which is the common practice in soap making. Superfatting at 5% makes soap feel more luxurious and moisturizing without inhibiting lather or making it too soft.

You can definitely super fat your soap at a higher percentage – some soap makers even go up to 15%. However, soaps with more oils are prone to have dreaded orange spots (DOS), which are usually caused by oils that have gone rancid.

You don't have to make any changes under Soap qualities and fatty acids since this is for more experienced soap makers who want to create their own recipe. What you need to do is select the oils you'll be using from Oils, Fats, and Waxes.

Each time you select an oil, press the Add button under Recipe Oil List. If you make a mistake and have to remove oil from the list, press the Remove button. You can also add and remove an item by pressing "+" and "-" buttons.

The two rightmost columns allow you to choose how you want to express the amount of oil in your recipe—either by percentage or the actual weight.

Whichever you choose, enter the amount of oil you'll be using.

When you're done listing all the oils, press the Calculate Recipe button. The Totals row will be automatically filled. The values should be equal to 100 and the amount you entered under Weight of Oils.

Click the View or Print Recipe button. This will display a table showing the amounts of water and lye that you should use.

Chapter 9: Soap Making Mold - Let Your Imagination Run Wild

In making bar soaps, using a soap making mold is quite necessary. You cannot complete your soap making process without pouring your liquid soap into a mold. And since it is an essential part of your process of making soap, why not make this step a very exciting one to highlight your experience.

There are countless molds to choose from. There are those which are readily available in crafts stores or even hardware stores. But there are soap making mold that can also be found inside your house. Yes, you read me right...in your own house. Practically anything that can hold a liquid mixture can be a soap mold. You just have to be creative in looking at things. Take for instance a wooden salad spoon. The deeper the spoon, the better it is.

I can attest to the flexibility of this famous kitchen utensil because I used it once as a soap making mold. I was in a rush to attend a simple all-girls night out with former high school classmates. And I wanted to use this opportunity to give out samples of my homemade soap. I was just starting with my business and I want to get as many prospects as possible. So I thought why not use the occasion to my advantage.

But I don't have a readily available mold and I can't leave the house to buy. So a sparkling idea came to mind. Why not use what is within my reach? And the first thing I saw, since I was in the kitchen preparing dinner, is my salad spoon. The shape is oval and the material is perfect because then if I will only put a parchment paper before pouring the soap mixture, I can easily take out the molded soap.

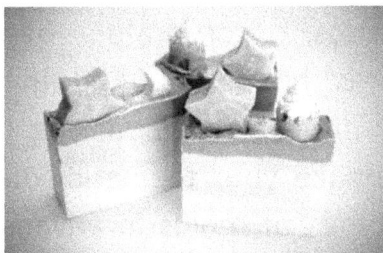

I also tried using a plastic cup. The shape can be unexciting but I put some hand painted decoration to put some character into the soap. I also saw a heart-shaped silicone container. I am not sure for what purpose is this, but I saw it kept somewhere so I thought that perhaps it can also be used as a soap making mold. And viola! The soap turned out to be a great gift.

When it comes to making soap, you can let your imagination run wild. And one easy way to do this is to be creative with the choice of soap making mold to use. You can even make a thematic set of soap for any occasion. It can be a great party give-away. Weddings, birthdays, christening, anniversaries, corporate events...the occasion is boundless. And if you are seriously into the soap making business, you can make your thematic soaps using various types of molds in advanced. And you can just keep them for future orders. Just remember to secure them tight so you don't lose the quality of your homemade soap.

Use Up Your Free Time With Soap Making

If you seem to have some free time at home and feel bored, then a new hobby that you can try taking up is soap making. It is not only very fun, but it is also a practical hobby to try as you will be able to make use of your soap once you are done. It is also easy to start as the materials and ingredients that you will need are very easy to acquire.

You will only need oil and lye as your main ingredients to make your soap. In addition to these, you will also need pails, mixing bowls and tools, molds and knives. With just these few equipment, you will already be able to start making soap that you can use in your bathroom.

Other than these basic ingredients and tools, you may also want to have coloring dyes and fragrant oils so that you can choose what color your soap will be, and how it smells like. You may also add lotions or herbal extracts to your soap to give them added properties. Lastly, changing the type of oil that you will use will also have a big difference on how your final soap turns out.

You may also want to do some research on how you will go about making your soap. There are two ways as to how to produce soap, one is through the hot process while the other is through the cold process. The entire process will not take more than an hour and after this, you will just be waiting until your soap has hardened on your molds.

Due to the ease of soap making, even small children can take this up as a hobby. One thing that you should change when kids are making soap is discarding the use of lye and instead, use glycerin soap. Glycerin soap is already prepared and children will not have to handle lye which is very dangerous especially without adult supervision.

This hobby is great for helping children develop their creative minds as they will think of creative ways of how to design their soaps. It is a better alternative than just letting your children stay at home and watching television all day. This might even be an exciting experience for them especially when they are going to use their soaps in the bathroom.

After making your soap, the most obvious thing to do with them next is use them in the bathroom. But aside from this, you may also want to just use them as bathroom decors especially if you were able to make a great design. These are also great as gifts or you may want to sell them if you become really great at making them.

Soap making is a very easy and practical hobby that is really worth trying. It won't take a lot of time to do so if you didn't enjoy it, you may move on to try other hobbies. But if you really enjoyed making soap, it is a hobby that would keep you busy for a very long time.

Soap Making and Its Advantages in Our Lives

People have already made the wise decision of switching to organic beauty products. Chemicals used in these products may harm the skin when used. Particularly for soaps, we use them on a daily basis so we have to make sure that the product that we are using is safe on the skin.

The art of soap making is indeed an interesting activity that you should try out.

This allows you to make organic soaps that are safe for the skin. You do not have to worry about your skin drying as well as getting allergies and rashes. All of the ingredients that you will use are practically natural so there is no need to worry about these anymore. Everything that you are looking for in a safe soap to use can be found in these kinds of soaps.

Soap is practically made through the process of saponification. It is practically the hydrolysis of fatty acid esters with a base to form the carbolyxate soaps. In simple terms, you just have to mix animal or vegetable oil with lye to form your soaps. This is how simple soaps are made. You can definitely enjoy this activity as you make soaps that you can actually use.

Start soap making by the easiest method-the 'melt and pour' method. This type of soap making method is actually very simple to follow. All that you have to do is buy the soap base. It just has to be melted before you add any of the additives for the soap. Once it has created a homogenous mixture, you can now have the soap harden. As soon as it does, you can start using what you made.

The secret to having an effective soap is picking the right natural oils to use for it. Top choices for these are coconut oil, palm oil and olive oil. The advantage of using these in your soaps is that it cleanses the body without drying up.

You can rely on your creativity if you really want to make beautiful soaps. There are a lot of molds that you can use for soaps. These come in different shapes and sizes. You can take a visit to your favorite hobby store or even pick up a baking pan. You can even buy cookie cutters to cut out the soaps that you have made. It is all up to you on how you want to decorate your soaps.

Soap making is not just an activity that you can play with. Since you are handling dangerous raw materials, you have to make sure that you have protective covering. Never handle lye without the proper safety gear such as goggles, apron and even gas mask.

Organic handmade soaps are very fun to use! Especially if you made them from scratch, you will definitely enjoy using them. Switch to the safer alternative when using soaps. Do not let your skin get harmed. If you want beautiful skin, switch to only the natural choice.

Try Soap Making As a New and Interesting Hobby

When you go into hotels, do you notice those specially made soaps that make their bathrooms extra attractive? Or have you seen soaps that are displayed in specialty stores? These soaps may seem really hard to make and you might think that these require special equipment and machinery to make. But contrary to what you may think, soap making is an easy process that you can do at home.

Soap is made from a fairly easy process called saponification. It is basically done by mixing the two basic ingredients in water and letting them undergo a reaction that will produce soap. And if you think these two ingredients are very hard to find, think again as you will only need some fats and lye and you can already start with your soap making process.

The first method of saponification is the hot process. This requires heating of the lye and water solution, and upon addition of the fats, further heating is still required. This method is used if you have an impure lye and don't have its exact amount. The quality of soap produced in this process may not be as good as the cold process but it can serve its purpose of cleaning.

The second method of saponification is through the cold process. This process will not require heating of the fats and lye mixture, instead it relies on the heat produced by mixing lye in water. The catch in this method is that you have to follow the exact amounts of each ingredient or you will not be able to produce a good type of soap. You will need pure lye in order to achieve the desired results.

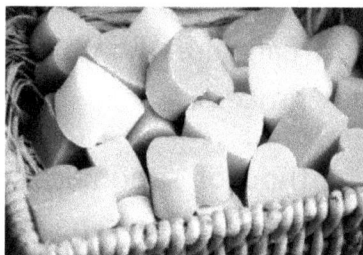

The first step in to making those soaps with advanced designs is by first mastering the basics. You will need to learn how to make soap that has the properties that you need by changing the type of fat you use, as well as the exact amounts that you will need. Once you have mastered how to make the basic soap, you can then move on to making more advanced designs.

The ingredients that you will need to make more advanced soaps are dyes and fragrances. In addition to these, you may also need several molds and a knife which can be used for sculpting soap. Dyes will of course give you the color of the soap that you want, and fragrances will add to the appeal of your soap. Molds and knives will help you shape your soap in any way that you please.

But soap making is not all fun and games. You must also be careful as lye is a very corrosive substance. It also emits dangerous fumes when immersed in water. This is why you should take precautions such as wearing gloves and face masks in order to protect yourself from its harmful effects.

Keep on practicing and eventually, you will start coming up with soaps that are comparable to those that you see in specialty shops and hotel bathrooms. One day, you might even surpass their designs and you may want to sell your own designs and earn some money from this hobby.

Herbal Soap Making - Are You Treating Your Skin to the Best Soap?

Isn't it better to use natural soaps rather than those with a lot of chemicals? Your beautiful skin deserves that natural treat too, so try using herbal soaps. Or why not start herbal soap making at home? This is so much better, right? - Enjoying the benefit of an all-natural body soap and having fun at the same time.

What is herbal soap? They are soaps that are mixed with natural ingredients such as juice, extract, or even chopped leaves of herbal plants. Herbal are safe to use except for those excessively sensitive skin, they should be vigilant for herbs that may irritate them.

Making herbal soaps are generally similar with other soap making process, what makes them distinctive to other process is the adding and choice of herbs incorporated into the soap. What are the herbs that are best used in soaps? Mint is a good choice for everyday soap that gives the user that invigorating effect while lavender is best for a soothing fragrance that a lady may desire. For herbs that provide the whitening effect on the skin, choose herbs such as papaya, kalamansi, or kamias.

Guava and akapulko may give the medicinal benefits for anti-fungal or antiseptic properties. Avocado and cucumber are one of the best herbal beauty soaps. Once the herbs to be used are selected it is time to start making your first ever herbal soap.

Choose the herbs that you want, more so, combining different herbs helps in producing something different and something unique. Experimenting is the key to a new found soap combination which is what herbal soap making is all about. It is quite challenging but also exciting to do.

The soap making procedure

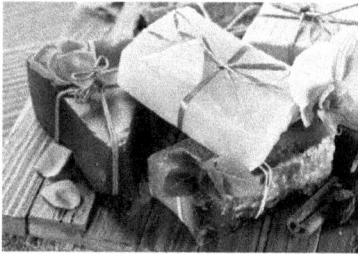

Prepare 1/4 cups of water and bring to a boil and add the herb of your choice, about 2 tablespoons of finely ground herbs. Let it steep for fifteen minutes.

Pour in the steeped mixture into a double boiler then reheat.

Add the soap which has already been cut into pieces and melt. Coloring and essential oils may also be added at this time to make your soap more attractive.

Once the mixture and the soap have completely mixed and totally melted, pour the soap into the mold and let it harden at room temperature. Coat the mold with vegetable oil before pouring the mixture in order to remove soap from mold easily.

After a few hours check if the soap has already hardened and remove from the mold.

Do not use the soap yet, let it cure for another day or two.

Herbal soap making is so simple, with the proper herbs and the skill to make the soap and presto...your new handcrafted soap!

Chapter 10: Fragrances

For many people, the fragrances are the most interesting part of the soap making process. In fact, many people like to really play around with fragrances in order to develop soaps that smell like very intriguing things, such as popcorn for example! But of course, if you are only just starting out with your soap making talents, you should stick to the idea of using scents to make your soap smell lovely and refreshing, and keep the experimental scents for a later date when you have some more experience making soap.

There are two ways to add scent to your soap. You can either do it with the help of essential oils, or you can do it with fragrance oils. Which one you choose to use depends on what you want the final properties of your soap to be, and how strong you want the scent to be as well.

Essential oils are very easy to use, and they are also very affordable. They come in all kinds of scents and different quantities, and they can be shipped from all over the world. They are usually the choice for people who want their soap to have a very natural smell. This is because they are actual plant and flower extracts, which means that they will not be enhanced beyond their own possibilities.

However, there is one problem that you will face if you decide to use essential oils. This is the fact that the scent will fade over time. The longer you store the soap bar without using it, the weaker the scent of the essential oils will be. This is often problematic for people who want to sell their soaps, because the customer will not be pleased if the soap bar doesn't have the scent that has been promised from the title. The scents that fade the fastest are those from citrus fruits. So, if you decide to make soap bars with this scent, make sure that you plan on using the soap as soon as possible.

On the other hand, fragrance oils are very different in this respect. They are the ones that are used in commercial perfume production, which is why you can expect them to last for years without fading. Of course, the quantities that are used in perfumes are much higher than those used in soap bars, but the scent will still remain for much longer than if you were to use essential oils.

Also, fragrance oils come in far greater varieties than essential oils. Because they are chemically produced, the production companies that make them can come up with virtually any scent that you can possibly think of. If you want your soap to have a smell that does not come directly from a plant or a flower, then you have to use fragrance oils by default because it will be the only way to produce this specific scent of your choosing.

However, the biggest problem with fragrance oils is that they are often the worst possible choice for people who suffer from sensitive skin or allergies. Most of these fragrance oils are patent protected, which means that you will never know the secret ingredients or the quantities of these ingredients that went into making a fragrance oil. This is a problem because without knowing the specific ingredients you cannot possibly easily market the product to a wider range of customers, since you cannot guarantee that your soap bar will not have an ingredient that your customer is allergic to. This of course becomes a very dangerous situation that you are much better off not having to deal with.

If you are just starting out and you don't want to deal with anything that could ruin the creativity of making soap, then you are much better off sticking to essential oils and the simplest possible ingredients that you can find. This will protect both you and the people who use your soap from having to deal with an unpleasant experience.

Scent Fixers

This process is a very interesting chemical one that helps to make the smell of essential oils last longer than they would normally be expected to last. Depending on what your final goal is, sometimes you can prolong the scent by adding another essential oil to the mix, while at other times you can fix the problem by adding an additive that will help your recipe be the best that it can possibly be. Of course, it is always best to stick to natural ingredients without additives, but if you are looking to become a professional soap maker, then you need to know as much as possible about the entire soap making process.

Below are some of the most popular fixers for soap recipes and how they contribute to the soap making process.

Arrowroot

This is a special root that comes from tropical plants. It is used in all kinds of cooking, which makes it safe for soap use as well. Its purpose is to thicken a mixture, but also to help the smell of the essential oil stick to the oil molecules of arrowroot, which will make the scent last much longer.

Benzoin

This oil has a number of different properties. It is most famous for being anti-inflammatory and antifungal, which makes it perfect for soap because you can use it to help ensure that your product will be even safer for use. Likewise, it is also a great ingredient for very dry and damaged skin, which means that you can add another healthy benefit to your soap recipe with this particular ingredient.

Corn starch

This ingredient doesn't really have any health benefits. Its main purpose has always been to help bind all of the ingredients together and to add an extra layer of thickness to the soap mixture that you are making. It could be a good ingredient to add if your mixture is very specific but also much thinner than you expected it to be. However, if you do decide to use corn starch, make sure that you mix it into the ingredients very well because it is notorious for leaving behind white bubbles that will ruin the look of your soap.

Oatmeal

The skin benefits of oatmeal are well-known and practically endless for people who have very sensitive skin. By adding it to your soap mixture, you will ensure that the oat milk that comes from this ingredient adds a new layer of moisture to your soap. However, you can also add finely milled oatmeal to add a bit of a scrub feature to your soap bar. It is an entirely natural ingredient that will not cause any discomfort for anyone who decides to use it.

Orris root powder

This is a great ingredient that will bring many benefits to the skin. It will help to add a layer of antioxidants to the skin and help to cleanse pores. It also has a very distinct smell of wood, which is lovely, but it is not one that is recommended to be used with other scents because it is likely to overpower them.

Essential oils

Another great way to lock in a scent and make sure that it lasts longer is to add another essential oil to the mix. You need the oils because the scent will stick to them the best, and thus it will help to keep your soap looking and feeling natural, while at the same time also helping it to smell lovely.

Soap Colors

Colors help to bring out the various varieties and beauties of soap bars. You can make an endless variety of designs with many colors to choose from, which will make the entire process of making soap very creative. There are many different sources from which you can get the different colors that you need from your designs. Some of these are artificial colors, while others are colors that are extracted from plants and flowers. In fact, you can even create your own colors from the flowers that you can grow in your own home or garden. However, this process is just slightly more complicated, so it is better to develop your own colors later on when you are more comfortable with the process of making soap.

Which color you use and where the color comes from will have a large effect on how your soap design will turn out in the end. Some colors are more dramatic than others. Natural colors usual give a natural color to the soaps, which is great because they don't add any artificial chemicals while at the same time providing a very beautiful natural color. There are a number of different sources from which you can extract colors, and we will list them below. However, as is the case with everything else, it is best to stick to the least difficult options while you are still in the process of learning how to best develop your own soap bars.

Oils

Some oils that you choose as part of your usual soap ingredients will have their own color. For example, olive oil will have a green hue, while oatmeal will have a creamy one. You can use a combination of the oils that would go into your recipe anyway to provide a natural color to your soap. This is one of the best ways for beginners to add color to their soap recipe without ruining the structure or the health benefits of the soap that they are making.

Clay

Clay is another natural ingredient that can be used to alter the color of your soap bars. Usually, there are not that many colors to choose from, but they are all natural and they have enough color to complete the design of any kind of soap that is made by beginners. Likewise, clay can also add a bit of a rough texture to the soap which would help to turn it into a bit of an exfoliant.

Minerals

The good thing about this source of color is that they come in almost any color that you can possibly imagine. However, although you would consider minerals to be natural, many people consider them not to be so. Although minerals are found in nature, they are often combined with other chemicals in order to make them have a specific color, which some think makes them not natural and harmful for the skin. These are similar minerals that you would find in makeup products, so if you don't mind using them in your soap go ahead but do keep in mind that you should not use them in soap recipes that are intended for sensitive skin.

Sugar

As you know, caramel is made when sugar is heated up and cooked at a specific temperature. The more you cook sugar, the deeper the caramel color will become. You can use this same technique to add a caramel color to your soap bar. In order to do this, you would cook the sugar separately and then carefully add it when you are ready. Likewise, if you add a rough texture of sugar in the soap bar, you can once again create the effect of a scrub.

Flowers, Herbs and Roots

Of course, whenever possible, the best ingredients to use in your soap recipes are the ones that come from nature. They are not only beautiful, but they are also the least likely to cause any kind of harm to the human skin. There is an endless number of colors that you can extract from nature, especially from flowers and herbs. Some people use things as simple as spinach or red onion skin in order to give color to your soap. You can freely become as creative as you want to be with this natural coloring process, because you will not be causing any harm to anyone using the soap. Also, you can become creative and free with your imagination.

Chapter 11: Scrub Bars

What Is a Scrub Bar?

A scrub bar is a type of body wash that can be likened to a mixture of body scrub and a bar of moisturizing bar soap. Rather than use a body scrub before cleaning up with a bar of soap, you can use a scrub bar to do both at a go!

Sugar Scrub Bars

The ingredients required for the making of these easy natural homemade sugar scrub bars are quite a few, and they might even be in your home right now. Basic silicone mould of any shape can be used for this scrub bar production process. It will be nice to have these sugar scrub bars in your bathroom, what would be nicer is giving them out as gifts to family and friends. In addition to saving cash and time in the shower, these sugar scrub bars also aid in the easy exfoliation of the skin. And exfoliation is a wonderful way of keeping the skin looking radiant and feeling soft, and these sugar scrub bars are a combination of skin-nourishing and gentle exfoliation ingredients such as glycerin, coconut oil, and lavender oil. These scrub bars are quite easy to make, and as such, it should earn a permanent spot in your shower and bath!

A Note About Ingredients

Before we delve further into how to make a sugar scrub bar yourself, I will like to give more insights and additional information regarding a couple of the ingredients that are listed in the recipe below. Firstly, you will be using a melt and pour method of soap making for the making of this scrub bar, and you are at liberty to choose a soap base of your choice! However, if you are not sure which of the soap base to melt and use, I will recommend an oatmeal soap base because of its skin-soothing characteristics and creamy texture. Secondly, if you are not familiar with a coloured mica, it is a sparkling mineral-based colourant that is used in the production of cosmetics and soap. The addition of mica to the ingredient is quite an easy way of adding shine and colour to sugar scrub bars, but adding a coloured mica is optional, and you can decide not to use it.

Tools and Supplies

Apart from the ingredients listed below, here is a list of the tools and/or supplies that will be needed to produce your own sugar scrub bars:

Silicone soap mould;

A small bowl;

A microwave-safe glass measuring cup;

Bamboo skewers.

Ingredients:

1 of cup sugar;

¼ cup of coconut oil;

½ cup of soap base for melt & pour;

15-20 drops lavender essential oil;

1 Tablespoon of vegetable glycerin;

Coloured mica (optional).

Instruction:

Start by cutting the melt & pour soap base into smaller pieces, then weigh out a heaping ½ cup of the soap base. Proceed by placing the soap base cubes inside a microwave-safe glass measuring cup and keep in a safe area.

Get the small bowl and pour the vegetable glycerin into it. If you are going with the mica, add it and stir the mixture very well with the bamboo skewer. The amount of mica you will add to the mixture is dependent on how radiant you want the scrub bar to be, and it is recommended that you start with ½ teaspoon, you can add more if needed.

Place the soap base in a microwave and heat it in 10-second increments, until it melts fully. Pour the coconut oil into the already melted soap base and stir it evenly till they both dissolve in each other. Proceed by adding sugar to the soap and oil mixture and resume stirring again.

Finally, pour in the glycerin mixture, essential oils and continue stirring with the bamboo skewer. After a while, the mixture will reach a light trace, at this point just place it in the microwave for another 10 seconds.

Pour the trace into the silicone mould and keep it in a safe area. Give the scrub bars 24 hours to solidify completely before removing them from the mould.

Shower Scrub Bars

Shower scrub bars are solid bars that are made from the wonderful cocoa butter and shea butter. This scrub bar moisturizes and exfoliates all the same time. Use one of these scrub bars in the shower and come out with silky, glowing and soft skin. The good news here is that you can easily make your own shower scrub bars in the comfort of your home with just a few ingredients. Here is the recipe for this uplifting shower scrub bar produced with shea butter and cocoa butter to help moisturize the skin, the Epsom salts exfoliate and lemongrass essential oil aid uplift and refresh the skin (this also boost blood circulation around the body).

Ingredients:

15g of shea butter;

55g of cocoa butter;

15g of vegetable oil of your choice (peach kernel, sunflower, fractionated coconut oil, etc.);

14g of almond wax or beeswax;

1g (approximately 20 drops) of lemongrass essential oil (or any other essential oil you prefer);

100g of coarse sea salt or Epsom salt;

Silicone ice cube tray.

Instruction:

Measure out the wax, jars of butter and vegetable oil, melt them together in a large stainless steel pot by placing the pot on a stove burning with medium heat.

Once everything has melted together, remove from the heat, proceed to mix the melted oils with the Epsom salt and essential oil. Stir until all the components dissolve in each other. Use a spoon or spatula to scoop the mixture and place it in the silicone mould.

Place the silicone mould in a refrigerator or freezer and give the bars 24 hours to set. Take one with to the shower and rub gently on your skin circular motions and rinse off. Come out of the shower with silky soft and glowing skin

Because shower scrub bars do not have a preservative, these are meant for one-time use only. This is why it is advisable to place them in a silicone ice cube tray; this way, they come out as the perfect size for one-time use.

Citrus-Rose Sugar Scrub Bars

Citrus-rose sugar scrub bars do not contain soap, so they do not lead to dry skin after use, unlike some sugar scrub bars. In addition, essential oils, shea butter, and beeswax are used for the production of these scrub bars and all these ingredients aid in moisturizing even the driest of skin.

Another plus for this scrub bar is that it holds the shape through hot showers and do not make a mess by turning oily. I highly advise that you make as many as possible, stash them for the next time you need a moisturizer and a polish ahead of a new season. Since these scrub bars hold their shape, they tend to last longer than other scrub bars as such you do not waste any. And this recipe given in this book will make a ton, so you have more than enough to keep in case of emergencies. When it comes to making sugar scrub, it is imperative that the bar is able to moisturize and exfoliate at the same time. So a combination of shea butter and essential oils are added to the recipe in bids to help lock in moisture and rejuvenate skin.

Also, if you have access to it, sweet orange oil comes in highly recommend. Not only is the smell amazing, but it is a wrinkle-fighting, anti-ageing powerhouse. Just a few drops of this oil is enough to help remove free radicals, improve cell growth and reduce inflammation. But in the absence of orange oil, kindly use any oil you have as the substitute. I am quite sure they will also give skin tons of benefits. Furthermore, dry skins need extra nourishment, as such, a big pinch of beetroot powder is included in the recipe, although this is optional beet powder is filled with vitamin C and A that brightens the skin and promote cell regeneration. Beet powder is not hard to find; there is a high chance that you will find it in the food sections at food stores nearest to you.

Ingredients:

1 cup of caster sugar;

1 teaspoon of beetroot powder;

1/3 cup of coconut oil;

¼ cup of beeswax granules;

1 ½ tablespoon of shea butter;

30 drops of sweet orange essential oil;

1 tablespoon of rose petals.

Muffin tin lined with paper or normal silicone moulds can be used to hold the scrub bar after production or paper-lined muffin tins.

Instructions:

Measure out the beeswax, shea butter, and coconut oil, melt them together in a large stainless steel pot by placing the pot on a stove burning with medium heat. Until everything is melted, then use a stick blender to whisk.

Add the beetroot powder, essential oil, and rose petals, and stir again.

Gently pour the sugar in and stir the mixture together till you get a medium trace. If you have a hard time with the mixture becoming thick too fast, just place the mixture in the microwave and heat for another 30 seconds.

Scoop the mixture into the soap moulds and place in the freezer for 20 to 30 minutes to cool. For use, rub the scrub in your palms to warm it when you notice a slight melt in your hands, buff the skin gently before rinsing it with water.

Body Scrub Cubes with Green Tea and Ginger

As opposed to popular opinion, it is not only the cold months of winter that wreak havoc on the human skin. Summertimes can also have devastating effects of irritation and dry skin, especially if you have spent several hours basking in the sun at the pool or beach. According to the information released by a national online survey in 2015 more than one thousand women over the age of 18 reported that as they grow older, the more difficult it is becoming to keep the skin moisturized. This is where an excellent combination of body scrub and a therapeutic moisturizer come into play. These homemade body scrub cubes are filled with ingredients that will soothe your skin, ingredients such as green tea, coconut oil, and ginger will cleanse and also rejuvenate the skin you have soaked in the summer sun. And because they are kept in a freezer, these body scrub bring along an extra cooling effect to calm your skin and promote healing. The use of coffee that is freshly ground to exfoliate makes it possible to avoid the harshness of sugar, which sometimes worsen irritation and redness.

Ingredients:

2 teaspoons of ground ginger;

2 tablespoons of loose green tea;

½ cup of coconut oil;

½ cup of fresh coffee grounds (un-brewed).

Instructions:

Add the green tea to the melted coconut oil in a small saucepan and place over low heat for 30 minutes. Let it cool for 20 minutes after removal from the heat. Use a fine-mesh strainer to remove the tea leaves from the oil and throw them in the trash. Add coffee grounds and ginger to the oil, stir it until all the components are properly mixed. Scoop the mixture into a silicone ice cube trays and freeze until it turns rock solid. It is advisable to use them in the shower and ensure your entire body is thoroughly rinsed to feel the full effect on the skin.

Homemade Sugar Scrub Bars for Dry Skin

It is quite difficult to keep dry skin well moisturized, but these homemade sugar scrub bars get the job done efficiently. And they also do it in style. Produced with a strong combination of coconut oil, shea butter, brown sugar, and cacao butter, in a recipe that will leave your skin hydrated and soft. The recipe stated below will yield 6 scrub bars

Ingredients:

Brown Sugar Stripes

1 tablespoon of coconut oil;

¼ cup of cocoa butter;

Silicone mould;

¼ cup of shea butter;

Small microwave-safe bowl;

1 cup of brown sugar.

Shea Butter Stripes

1 tablespoon of honey;

¾ cup of cocoa butter;

2 tablespoons of coconut oil;

¾ cup of shea butter;

15 drops of bergamot essential oil.

Instructions:

Brown sugar scrub bar

Place the shea butter, cocoa butter and coconut oil inside a stainless steel pot, place on a stove burning at minimum heat until all the oils and butter melts completely.

Add the brown sugar to the oil and stir very well until it dissolves into a sandy texture, not soupy or runny. You can add more sugar if necessary.

Scoop the mixture inside a silicon mould. Place in the freezer until it turns rock solid.

Shea butter scrub bar

Add the ¾ cup of cocoa butter, 2 tablespoons of coconut oil and ¾ cup of shea butter in a clean bowl, place on a stove burning at minimum heat until all the oils and butter melts completely

Add the bergamot oil and honey and stir till evenly mixed.

Leave the mixture to cool for 25 minutes. Then scoop the mixture inside a silicon mould. Place in the freezer until it turns rock solid.

You can unmold the scrub bars from the silicon mould, store the scrub bars in a container that is airtight in the freezer until you need it again.

Pet Shampoo

Having a pet is quite an expensive activity as a pet owner is saddled with feeding the pet, buying toys, safety gears and periodic checkups for the dog. As a matter of fact, keeping a pet happy and healthy can sometimes feel like you are taking care of a child! However, being a pet owner does not mean you have to exhaust your finances by doing all of your shopping at the local pet store. Take the hygiene of the pet for instance, why waste cash on shampoos bought from stores when you can produce your own? If you have it at the back of your mind that producing natural homemade dog shampoo will be difficult, you better think again because not only does it take a few minutes to produce your own natural homemade shampoo, the shampoo making process also require a handful of day to day ingredients you most likely have in the pantry already.

Irrespective of maybe you like to use natural products for your pet, or you are a regular do it yourself kind of person or better still, you want to save some cash! Producing your own dog shampoo is a way of achieving all three. Guess what! The ingredients may be lying idle on your shelf, and if it is not there, you can easily source from them in the nearest store. All you need are basic ingredients such as vinegar, ordinary dish soap, and vinegar. One thing you should avoid at all costs is using human shampoo for pets. The level of pH of the human skin is different from the pH level of the dog's skin – healthy human pH range for skin is 4.5 to 6.5, while dogs' healthy range is between 6 and 8.5. As a result of this, shampoo meant for humans is too acidic for dogs and can lead to irritation on the skin. If you are planning to make your own dog shampoo, you should be targeting a pet shampoo with a pH level of around 7. That is a lot of chemistry, isn't it? Well, as fate would have it, some people have already done the calculations for you and came up with simple recipes for homemade dog shampoos. Remember to use ingredients that will have a pH level around the 7 marks. The majority of soap bases and soaps will have their pH levels written on the label.

The pHs of some basic items used for pet shampoos:

Water: 7.0 (neutral - neither acidic nor alkaline);

Baking Soda: 8.3 (alkaline);

Lemon Juice: 2.0 (acid);

Vinegar: 2.2 (acid).

When you add these basic ingredients together to produce a dog shampoo, make sure you are balancing acidic substance like lemon juice with an alkaline substance such as baking soda in a base that is neutral (water) in bids to make sure the pH of the shampoos will not lead to any irritation on the skin of the dog. Too much alkaline does not pose a threat, but too acidic will cause skin irritation and can even burn the skin of the dog.

The recipes I will mention in this book will give you the ultimate homemade dog shampoo that will save you money and time, but most essentially, this shampoo will make your dog smell fresh and look clean. If you have normal dishwashing detergent and vinegar in your kitchen, you are good to go as you have the basic ingredients needed to make a powerful homemade dog shampoo.

Every pet needs a regular bath, even dogs that hardly shed need to bath regularly. When the topic is about how to clean your dog, there are many relatively cheap, gentle and natural ways of cleaning your pet. Homemade dog shampoo is holding the key for the lock you seek.

What is not green about commercial dog shampoos?

Some of the ingredients used for the production of commercial dog shampoos may sound catchy when we hear them, but in actual fact, they bringing more harm than good to the dogs as some of these ingredients can cause flakiness, discomfort, and itching when used on the sensitive skin of the dog. Some ingredients, however, do not sound nice from the get-go! An example is Polyethylene Glycol (PEG), which is a typical cosmetic base and is present in some shampoos mean for pets. This substance is a petroleum product that can remove the natural moisture of the skin. Sodium Lauryl Sulfate (SLS) and its variant - Sodium Laureth Sulfate (SLES), are ingredients commonly used in the production of some commercial dog shampoos, these substances can increase the risk of severe irritation of the skin, diarrhoea, and eye damage.

Several of the cosmetics and body care products used by humans are discarding the use of certain substances that can still be found in shampoos for dogs. Some of these substances include phthalates, that handles viscosity, or paraben, a preservative that is used to elongate the shelf life. While several of us are not so bothered about the application of these small dose chemicals when it is time for your pet to have its bathe, we should be concerned about the effect it is having on the skin of the dog.

Dish Detergent and Soap

Liquid soaps are commonly used to clean dirty dishes but what you do not know is that it is a wonderful ingredient when it comes to keeping your pet clean. Dish detergents are designed specially to clean out the grease with ease, and this means they are perfect for making a homemade dog shampoo because they can clean off oils that have accumulated oils on the coat and skin of your dog.

That is not all though. Dish detergent with lavender scent can also act as a flea repellant. So, bathing your dog occasionally in a homemade dog shampoo that contains these ingredients can aid in giving your dog a healthy lifestyle without you worrying about harmful chemicals present in commercial dog shampoos and without having to break the bank to take care of your pet.

Even if fleas are not disturbing your dog, the benefits to the skin are positive, and the scent of lavender will make the dog happy and smelling wonderful at the same time.

White Vinegar

Another wonderful ingredient in the dog shampoo is white vinegar. This basic household item is an excellent addition to the recipe for homemade dog shampoo due to its deodorant and antibacterial properties. When added to the dish detergent in the recipe for your homemade dog shampoo, the final product will make the coat of the dog shiny and healthy and shiny, while also giving antibacterial protection.

A quick word of WARNING - white vinegar is slightly acidic in nature. Since it will be added to the recipe of your homemade dog shampoo, it is advisable to be extremely careful when using it around the face and eyes of the dog as it can cause a burning sensation for the pup.

The Ultimate Homemade Dog Shampoo Recipe

Since you have your white vinegar and dish detergent on the ground, all that is left is a spray bottle. The process of mixing these ingredients is quite simple and requires only three stages:

Pour two cups of warm water inside the bottle;

Pour ½ cup of white vinegar to the water in the bottle;

Pour ¼ cup of dish detergent to the mixture inside the bottle.

Once all the three-ingredient are inside the bottle, shake the bottle gently to combine the ingredients until you notice a layer of bubbles inside the bottle. Allow these bubbles to dissipate before using the shampoo.

When it is time for your dog to have it bathe, just wet the coat of your dog with warm water and apply the homemade dog shampoo mixture on every part of their body. Once the shampoo is poured on the coat of the dog, go ahead and give your dog a good massage and use your hands to make a rich, thick lather on their coat. It is recommended to be done this way because the mixture will get down to the skin and give an efficient washing up. To wrap up the bath, just rinse the shampoo of the fur of your dog and leave them to dry off. They will look clean and smell fresh after a few minutes.

Additional Homemade Dog Shampoo Recipes

Sensitive skin Dog Shampoo recipe:

1 quart of water (32 ounces);

2 tablespoons of aloe vera gel;

1 cup of apple cider vinegar or white vinegar;

1/3 cup of glycerin;

1 cup of nontoxic dish soap scented with lavender.

Puppies or small dog shampoo recipe:

1/4 cup of white vinegar or apple cider vinegar;

1/2 cup of water;

1/4 cup of nontoxic dish soap scented with lavender.

Dish detergent is created to cut through the grease with ease and will do a wonderful job of cleaning up oils that gather on the coat and skin of your dog. White vinegar has both deodorant and antibacterial properties and will make the coat clean and shiny. Just make sure you don't get any of these shampoos in the eye of the dog. Add all the ingredients in the recipe in a spray bottle and shake well to mix thoroughly. Then spray warm water on the coat of your dog and apply the shampoo avoiding the eyes. Use your hands to work the shampoo into a thick lather on the coat of the dog. Rinse it all off, dry up the dog and set the dog free!

Homemade Dog Shampoos for Dry Skin

If you notice that your pet has a dry, itchy, or sensitive skin, there are certain things that can be added to the shampoo to eliminate his symptoms. It is possible to produce a shampoo with glycerin and aloe vera gel as part of the ingredients. You can buy glycerin from pharmacies, grocery stores, and/or online. Or you can produce an oatmeal shampoo. Oatmeal is famous for its skin-soothing characteristics, and it is present in various commercial grooming products.

Ingredients:

1 quart of water;

1 cup of dish soap that is nontoxic or baby shampoo;

1 cup of apple cider or white vinegar;

1/3 cup of glycerin;

2 tablespoons of aloe vera gel.

Mix every ingredient in a spray bottle and shake to mix evenly. Spray it on your dog, avoiding the eyes and use your hand to work his coat. Rinse it all off and allow it to dry up.

Oatmeal Dog Shampoo for Dry Skin

Ingredients:

1 cup of uncooked oatmeal;

1 quart of warm water;

1/2 cup of baking soda.

Using a food processor or a coffee grinder to grind the oatmeal until it looks like flour. Pour into a big bowl, add baking soda and mix it together. Pour warm water and mix until it dissolves in each other. Wet the dog with warm water and then pour the natural homemade shampoo on the skin of the dog. Work for your hand on his coat and allow the shampoo to sit on the coat for a few minutes. Rinse thoroughly and dry the skin of the dog with a dry towel.

Homemade Shampoo to Repel and Kill Fleas

Homemade dog shampoo can even be used to fight fleas. The trick here is the addition of lavender essential oil to the recipe, and this essential oil is a natural antibacterial and anti-parasitic. Although you can add a variety of oils such as eucalyptus, peppermint, lavender, and rosemary if you have to pick only one, lavender is okay. You have to understand that it is not every essential oil that is acceptable. Some dogs will react negatively after exposure to some essential oils (for example, - potpourri). Do not use 100 per cent essential oils derived from aromatherapy products on the dog, especially if the dog has broken skin. Also, ensure that your dog does not ingest the essential oils.

Ingredients:

2 ounces of aloe vera gel;

10 ounces of warm water;

2 drops of lavender essential oil;

1 tablespoon of Castile soap.

Note: you can add 2 drops rosemary, eucalyptus, and peppermint essential oils.

Combine every ingredient in a spray bottle and shake vigorously to mix evenly. Spray warm water on the dog, then apply the shampoo and use your hands to work it into the coat of the dog, particularly for places that are quite hard to reach and avoid his eyes. Rinse it all off and dry the dog with a towel.

Homemade Dog Shampoo with Coconut Oil

The last homemade shampoo for dogs is the natural dog shampoo recipe with coconut oil. It is an open secret that coconut has a whole lot of benefits for your dog, but the oil can also act as a good moisturizer when added to a shampoo recipe.

Ingredients:

½ cup of castile soap;

¾ cup of distilled water;

¼ cup of coconut oil;

5 drops of lavender essential oil.

Combine every ingredient in a spray bottle and shake vigorously to mix evenly. Spray warm water on the dog, then apply the shampoo and use your hands to work it into the coat of the dog, particularly for places that are quite hard to reach and avoid his eyes. Rinse it all off and dry the dog with a towel.

There are tons of homemade recipes for dog shampoo recipes, but one thing common to most of them is use of vinegar, that add shine and deodorizes; dish soap or Castile soap, that aids in the binding together of the ingredients in the recipe; and baking soda that used to balance the acidity of water (neutral pH) and vinegar.

Essentials oils will also give an organic and nice touch, so when next you are making shampoo for your dog, begin in the kitchen and combine some safe, easy and relatively cheap shampoos of your own

Chapter 12: Soap For Sale

It's the day you've been waiting for! -The day when you're finally ready to sell your soap. Like all business's you need to make sure that you have your product ready which is home-made soap, pre-cut, wrapped and labeled with your company name. Here are some pointers on how to start getting you soap out there.

Samples

Making samples can be fun and easy to do. One way to go is to slice your soap into a few bars (whatever size or shape you like). Once they're package slide a business card in with the soaps or attach at the outside if possible. Some people even include information on how their soap is beneficial and can help improve your skin. Another way to go is to add a coupon with your sample. For example, buy 3 bars and get 3 more for free.

Targeting the people you know or the people you work with first is always a good idea and can help build up your confidence in your new soap business. Plus, people rarely pass up free products and if your soap is good they'll want more!

Market

Once you're comfortable sampling to the people you already know you'll want to try other places. A matter of where to sell your product can be difficult. Luckily, you have this guide to help you!

A great way to start is with flea markets, bazaars, or festivals. Renting a booth is usually pretty affordable depending on the event. Other than selling your soap make sure to give out plenty of business cards even to the people that didn't purchase any. This is a useful marketing strategy because that person will have it handy when they think they might actually need or want the soap.

First impressions last! Always keep your booth or table display presentable with plenty of products to show. Potential customers will rarely share what they're thinking so don't give them the opportunity to get the wrong idea. Having a price list is beneficial in this case as most shoppers will be too shy to ask or might have already made up their might on whether they can afford it or not.

Don't get lazy! Keep your energy up and be enthusiastic when building rapport with someone who approaches your booth. If a customer is already in doubt about your product seeing you sitting behind the booth entranced in your cell phone won't help. Let them know that your passion for your business is what makes your soap crafted to perfection with the best quality.

Never give up! First times can be rocky especially if marketing is new to you. Sales will increase over time so stick with it. Going to the same festivals or bazaars on a frequent basis will also increase your chance of customer coming back to buy the soap they took a sample of the previous week. Your loyal customer may even recommend your soap to others.

Online Marketing

People are shopping online for just about anything these days. Online Marketing has helped numerous businesses boom by simply having attractive advertising.

Building the website might sound painstaking and challenging but if you check online there are tons of user friendly site builders available. Be sure use one that's affordable and has good customer support.

Since this is a soap business I can't stress enough how important the pictures of your soap will be. Shoppers won't have the privilege of smelling the wonderful aromas and oils. The pictures will be a major selling point in attracting potential buyers. Of course the picture goes hand in hand with the description. Don't be afraid to go into detail about how the soap smells and feels. It's all about building a desire and imagery of having the soap already and loving it!

Be original! Pictures are important but nothing's worse than having fake pictures of soap that's not yours! Most shoppers will be able tell when they realize they've seen the same picture on Google images. How do you think your new customer will react when they get they're box of soap in the mail and see that it's not what they expected—bye bye customer loyalty!

Make it user friendly. Let's face it, not all of your customer's are going to be patient enough to have to search every link on your page for the shopping cart. Make it easy for them to place their order by having a clean and clear buying process. Create a Contact Us tab with a message box or phone number so they know they're buying home-made soap from a real person who cares about their interest.

Chapter 13: How To Ph Test Handmade Soap

pH is a measurement of the hydrogen ion concentration in an aqueous solution. Solutions with a high concentration of hydrogen ions have a low pH, while solutions with a low concentrations of hydrogen ions have a high pH.

One of the common questions that come up on Soapmaking is how to pH test handmade soap.

I hope to clear up a lot of common misconceptions about the why and how of pH testing handmade soap in this book, and will be including information and examples for various kinds of soap! Before we dive in, let's review…

What is pH ?

Neutral is a pH of 7, while anything above that is alkaline, and anything below is acidic. Most people are familiar with the pH of household substances like milk or various cleaning products, but just in case you aren't, here's a quick approximate comparison chart of common materials on a pH scale:

Handmade soaps are typically between a pH of 8 and 10.

As far as I'm aware , it is impossible for a handmade soap to fall near neutral or below without using an emulsifier to keep the soap molecules within the solution. I know that soapmakers frequently state that they can or do create neutral pH soap, but such products don't tend to be true soap, meaning that they aren't composed mainly of the alkali salts of fatty acids.

Important Notes about pH & Soap

There are two key points I want to jump into here, before we start talking about pH testing soaps.

First, it is important to keep in mind that pH is a measurement of hydrogen ions in an . It is not a measurement of hydrogen ions in substance you feel like measuring! Obviously, when you are looking at bar soap, it is a relatively solid material an aqueous solution. In order to properly test the pH of a bar soap, you should attempt to use a solution.

The second important note is that pH is not a direct relationship to how harsh or mild a product is.

What's the point of pH testing soap ?

First, unless a soap contains a large amount of excess alkali, it could test within a pH range for handmade soap (). And, if given enough time to cure, lye-heavy soap could eventually test normal as carbon dioxide works its magic onfree alkali.

Plus, handmade soap fresh out of the mold could be unfinished, in that saponification is not fully complete. How quickly a properly made soap saponifies depends on the oils used as well as the temperature of the soap and the environment, and can range from as little as 24 hours to multiple weeks.

The Do and Dont's of pH Testing Handmade Soap

If you do want to pH test your soap, it's important to start off on the right foot.

I know plenty of soapmakers who use this method in their process, and while I won't argue its efficiency or efficacy, I will argue it's safety. If a new soapmaker comes across this advice and has not yet familiarized themselves with the appearance of lye heavy soap, tongue testing could result in serious injury.

Using Tongue Testing or Zap Testing to Check Soap Alkalinity

An extremely common recommendation I found as a method of checking the soap pH is to touch a bar of soap to your tongue. If touching the bar of soap to your tongue zaps similar to touching your tongue to a battery, it indicates a soap is lye heavy. Obviously, this doesn't actually indicate the pH level of a soap, it simply indicates the presence of free alkali.

Just say "no" to tongue testing or zap testing!

Using pH Strips to Test Soap pH

That is the next most common method of pH testing soap .

Using pH strips directly on a bar of soap can give you an inaccurate pH reading that is so far off you might think your soap is neutral!

The first problem with pH strips is that the nature of soap interferes with the indicator dyes used to manufacture the strips, which can throw the reading off by several points.

The second issue is that the process of putting water on the surface and rubbing it until it lathers createsa huge variable. How much or how little soap is dispersed in the water can affect the reading of the pH.

If pH strips are all you've got and you are wildly curious about the pH of your soap, using a specific solution and higher quality pH strips will help get some of these variables under control. **Let's do not forget that using pH strips is not the most ideal method of checking a soap's pH.**

How to pH Test Handmade Soap

Now that we've talked about all the issues with pH testing soap, let's get down to business with how to pH test soap in the most ideal way.

First, boil distilled water, which will serve two purposes: help eliminate carbon dioxide and help dissolve the soap. Next, shave pieces of the soap from the side of the bar, from top to bottom, using a knife, into a clean disposable cup.

You are aiming for a 1% soap solution, meaning 1% of the solution is soap and 99% of the solution is distilled water.

Next, add the distilled water, with a temperature reading of about 70 C (), to a glass mason jar and then add the soap shavings. (stirr the solution until the soap dissolve

The standards mention that you should conduct the pH test at 40⁻ C (), which is about 104⁻ F and that the solution should be rapidly cooled.To do so,place your mason jar is an ice bath and keep an eye on the temperature while I preparing the pH testing materials.

Each one of the pH testing materials you will use come with varying levels of instructions for accurate readings, so you have to default to each individual one for instructions. For instance, some pH testing strips say to submerge the strip for 30 seconds while others say to dip the strip in the solution.

Whenever I teach a basic soap making class, the students are always super eager to jump right in and make a batch of soap right away! Many of the ingredients can be found locally or at the grocery store, and many more can be ordered online for quick delivery.

But let's say you aren't quite sure about this whole soap making adventure, and don't want to invest a lot of money into equipment. One of the biggest (and best) investments you'll make is in your soap mold. Here are some very inexpensive or no-cost soap molds that will get you started.

Chapter 14: Beginners Soap Making Mistakes

Regardless, making your first cluster of custom made cleanser isn't difficult to do. Apprentice cleanser committing errors help you take in more about making soap. Take after the headings, take as much time as is needed and read on the most proficient method to make custom made soap before attempting to make it.

At the point when the headings notice two thermometer's and a cleanser cutter, you better have them. I say this since I had neither one.

I committed the error of including my sodium hydroxide and water answer for my oil while they were both still too hot. Utilizing a hand blender accelerated the chilly cleaner process. I needed to empty the soap into my mold sooner than I ought to have.

Upon all the hurrying of emptying my blend into my mold. I neglected to include my essential oil and herb. I can not express my contemplations when I, at last, got my cleanser combination filled the molds and pivoted just to see my essential oil and herbs sitting on the counter.

At last in the wake of viewing a video on YouTube demonstrating to settle cleanser issues, my handcrafted soap turned out fine.

I was glad for my little measure of custom made soap. Making natively constructed soap is something I needed to do, and the inconvenience I experienced while making my first bunch was justified regardless of each mix-up and push to redress the oversights. I prescribe this distraction to anybody, and the prizes are incredible by only knowing it's your completed creation.

My second clump of handcrafted cleanser went incredibly after my involvement with my first group. My soap solidified and was prepared to cut. I didn't have a soap cutter. I requested a basic cleanser cutter which took more time for conveyance. My polish is hard to cut even with the soap cutter since I held up to long to cut the cleaner.

The bars were not equivalent in size, but rather I gave some of this cleanser to others and requested them to tell me how or if the soap helped their skin. This gives me a hand know what number of individuals could utilize soap with the organic oil and herbs I used as a part of Polish. Four did not answer but rather eighteen adored it.

The following are a few things I prescribe for learner cleanser producers to consider before bouncing into the task. I will concede my fledglings missteps to help ideally other people that are needing to figure out how to make hand crafted cleanser.

What you have to begin making icy procedure cleanser:

Security glasses and gloves

Cleaner Mold.

Cleanser cutter that functions admirably with the molds you have.

Wax paper or cooler paper.

One expensive stainless steel pot to blend the fixings. You can liquefy your strong cleanser oils in this, then include the liquid detergent oils. Lastly including the sodium hydroxide and water answer for the oils.

Two or more glass or plastic holders for your water and lye arrangement and liquid cleanser making oils. Measuring compartment function admirably.

Cleanser Formula

You may require more spoons and measure holders on the off chance that you are including shading, essential oils or herbs. Only lay your fixings out on your work territory and supply every fixing its particular compartment.

Fixings

Refined water

Sodium hydroxide

Cleanser oils and spreads you plan to use for your formula.

Herbs and any essential oils or hues you intend to use for the recipe.

My tips for Tenderfoot cleanser creators:

Never in solidness the sodium hydroxide arrangement.

Wear your security.

Use compartments with covers for the safety.

Have a lot of time to complete your cleanser making the venture.

Continuously utilize a cleaner number cruncher before using any soap formula.

Rehash the guidelines.

Temperatures for the sodium hydroxide and oil for frosty procedure cleanser are 95 - 100 degree Fahrenheit.

Continuously empty your dry sodium hydroxide into your water. Pouring gradually while mixing with a spoon constant until mixed.

Continuously pour your sodium hydroxide and water arrangement into your oils.

Know that utilizing a stick blender speeds up the cleanser making process. So know likewise of your dainty follow.

Continuously have two thermometers. One for the oils and the other for sodium hydroxide.

At the point when utilizing a little shape, you can use an expensive blade to cut the cleanser bars. At the point when utilizing an extensive section mold spend the additional cash to get the best possible cleanse cutter for the kind of image you are using, it's justified, despite all the trouble.

Cut your soap when it gets to be strong, more often than not around 24 hours. Holding up to long to cut your handcrafted soap makes the cutting procedure more troublesome, and results could be harmed cleanser bars.

At the point when requesting packs on the web, notice if the sodium hydroxide accompanies the unit or on the off chance that you need to purchase it elsewhere.

At the point when requesting cleanser making supplies dependable check the delivery cost.

All things considered, I had a ton of fun, and I adore my natively constructed lavender soap.

Conclusion

Having read this guide, you now have all the tools you need to make fabulous homemade soap. Unlike cooking where a few strange ingredients can make a horrific meal, soap making is all about experimentation. As long as you have the right amount of lye and fat you can let your imagination run wild and create some truly unique soap.

Don't be afraid of a soap turning out poorly – some of the most interesting effects will happen when you try out new things. The only danger you might run into is adding in new chemicals that speed up the sopanification process, however researching what you are putting in should give you a good indication of whether this will happen or not.

Making your own soap is one of the most rewarding of the home crafts you can take up because it gives you a luxury product that you can share with your friends and it really changes the way you view the cosmetics you use every day.

It's one of the easiest ways of applying your chemistry skills in real life and the obsession with making a perfect batch of soap can be inspiring.

Making the soap is just the beginning of your soap's life. People often want to start giving their soap away as gifts or selling them so there is a new range of things to consider.